Accession no
01081085

WITHDRAWN

D0718504

PREGNANT W...

WHAT MIDWIVES NEED TO KNOW

LIBRARY

Tel: 01244 375444   Ext: 330⁺

This book is to be
last date

Dedicated to

All our daughters in the hope that they may never be subjected to domestic violence; and for all our sons, hoping they never use violence as a source of communication.

And to

David Hunt and Kevin Martin for their support, patience and kindness and who by good luck are kind and gentle in all their ways.

Pregnant Women: Violent Men

What midwives need to know

Sheila C. Hunt and Ann M. Martin

141612I

CHESTER COLLEGE	
ACC. No. 01081085	DEPT.
CLASS No. 362·8292 HuN	
LIBRARY	

B*f*M Books *for* Midwives

OXFORD AUCKLAND BOSTON JOHANNESBURG MELBOURNE NEW DELHI

Books for Midwives
An imprint of Butterworth-Heinemann
Linacre House, Jordan Hill, Oxford OX2 8DP
225 Wildwood Avenue, Woburn, MA 01801-2041
A division of Reed Educational and Professional Publishing Ltd

℞ A member of the Reed Elsevier plc group

First published 2001

© Sheila C. Hunt and Ann M. Martin 2001

All rights reserved. No part of this publication may be reproduced in
any material form (including photocopying or storing in any medium by
electronic means and whether or not transiently or incidentally to some
other use of this publication) without the written permission of the
copyright holder except in accordance with the provisions of the Copyright,
Designs and Patents Act 1988 or under the terms of a licence issued by the
Copyright Licensing Agency Ltd, 90 Tottenham Court Road, London,
England W1P 0LP. Applications for the copyright holder's written
permission to reproduce any part of this publication should be addressed
to the publishers

British Library Cataloguing in Publication Data
A catalogue record for this book is available from the British Library

ISBN 0 7506 5203 9

Typeset by Avocet Typeset, Brill, Aylesbury, Bucks
Printed and bound in Great Britain by Biddles Ltd
www.biddles.co.uk

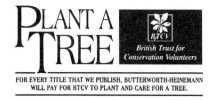

FOR EVERY TITLE THAT WE PUBLISH, BUTTERWORTH-HEINEMANN
WILL PAY FOR BTCV TO PLANT AND CARE FOR A TREE.

Contents

Chapter 4

Liberal feminism • Marxist feminism • Black feminism • Radical feminism • Patriarchal society • A continuum of male violence • Can feminism provide the answer to violence against women? • The power of the professional • Has professionalism benefited pregnant women?

Chapter 5

Why domestic violence in pregnancy? • The incidence of domestic violence in pregnancy • The changing nature of violence in pregnancy • Risk factors for domestic violence in pregnancy • Warning signs in the pregnancy history • The effects of abuse during pregnancy • After the birth of the baby

Chapter 6

So why does she stay? • Domestic violence: a case for midwifery intervention? • The use of direct questions, screening tools and assessment guides • So what can the midwife do? • Documentation. Dealing with photographic evidence • Barriers to intervention • Prevention of abuse of women? • Who can help the midwife? • Exploring professional responses • So how might the midwife act as an advocate and empower the abused woman?

Chapter 7

The Family Law Act 1996 • The Non-Molestation Order • Undertakings • Occupation Order • Enforcement: remand and arrest • The interaction with the Children Act 1989 • The Police • Why calling the police may not be the answer • Can the police help? • Domestic Violence Units • The Women's Aid network • Negative aspects of the Women's Aid and refuge provision – thinking the unthinkable.* • Treatment for the abuser and the abused

Chapter 8

The main issue • The Government response to domestic violence • The new NHS – modern and dependable • Making a difference • Back at the Trust.

Preface

Why do midwives need to know about violence against women? Why have we written this book? Obviously we feel that it is important that midwives and other health professionals offer women the best possible care. To this end, we believe that midwives should understand something of the complexities of domestic violence. Apart from the fact that no woman, midwife or not, can escape from the fear of violence, midwives also need to be aware of the ways in which they can intervene to change and possibly improve a battered woman's immediate and, perhaps, longer-term future. The idea that midwives can influence the experience of a pregnant woman in their care suggests that health professionals can exert a power over the outcome of their clients. Obviously, this is true if we think of the statutory authority given to social workers, or the decisions made by doctors on our behalf, but are midwives similarly powerful? Can they really do anything to change a woman's life? If they can, should they? Is it their role to intervene in a woman's life beyond their professional duties of supporting her through the medical and perhaps psychological processes of childbirth?

Throughout most of history, and still in many parts of the world today, midwives have been part of the social group they seek to serve. They have been part of the day-to-day life of local women, as well as part of the maternity care given to them. Sharing the lives of their pregnant neighbours, however, tended to relegate midwives' knowledge and skills. Their understanding of the links between women's social status and their health and pregnancies was ignored. They were seen as servants of society; a society in which women and their bodies were largely controlled by men (Hunt and Symonds, 1995). In this social context, the great midwife reformers of the late nineteenth and early twentieth centuries sought to focus attention on the plight of women of childbearing age. They rightly believed that the way to bring about social improvements was to gain recognition for the knowledge and skills of midwives by seeking professional status. In this way they believed that the voices of midwives would be heard, and that they would also give a voice to those seeking maternity care.

The thought that a woman could in some way be responsible for a violent attack on herself is, perhaps, the one idea that midwives and professionals need to rid themselves of. Whatever the circumstances, whatever the issues between couples, abuse is the unacceptable wielding of power by one person over another. As such, it is never acceptable or justified. It is this use of power, rather than the manifestation of it (that is, the actual violence) which must be acknowledged and challenged. The use (and abuse) of power is, however, not limited to intimate relationships. In this book we seek to examine the role of midwives in relation to childbearing women who are or have been abused. We want to consider how far the behaviour of professionals can either significantly help domestic violence victims, or victimise them further, and we want to offer practical steps to assist midwives in this aspect of their role.

Midwives hold a unique position of trust with the women they come into professional contact with. They can use this power positively, or they can abuse their position to undermine the right of autonomy of the pregnant woman. They can disclose information about her without her consent; they can trivialise what the woman is telling them; they can disbelieve her; they can blame the woman herself for the violence; and they can suggest that violence and abuse are normal features in many relationships. On the other hand, midwives can act as a sounding board for women in difficult times: they can show they believe and respect what is being told to them; they can show solidarity with their clients by acknowledging that no one deserves to be battered; they can have a knowledge of local community resources; above all they can demonstrate a complete acceptance of their client's right to make her own decisions, whether they agree with her or not. In this book we seek to help midwives to make a difference to some women's experience of childbirth. For the one in four women who are abused, we hope to make a difference.

Sheila C. Hunt
Ann M. Martin

Introduction

Domestic violence is most commonly described as the systematic abuse, both physical and mental, which takes place within the context of the family structure. The distinction between 'physical' and 'mental' abuse is both important and yet insignificant at the same time. It is important because it recognises that violence can encompass a far wider spectrum of bullying, humiliation and degradation than merely that which is inflicted by bodily assault. It is insignificant because abuse of one person by another is not mitigated by the means of that abuse, and therefore there is no real relevance to the distinction.

Domestic violence as a term can include such behaviour as physical, verbal or sexual assault, threats, taunting, belittling and, indeed, any other form of anti-social behaviour that is carried out over a period of time. Such acts form part of a complex and continuing pattern of behaviour, which is rooted in the power and domination of one individual over another.

Further consideration of the term domestic violence also highlights problems. It is important to ask these questions: 'Does it make sense to distinguish between domestic and other types of violence and why do we do so?'

Is it to suggest that violence within the confines of our 'safe' homes is considered far more unacceptable than 'ordinary' street violence committed randomly? Clearly not, when we realise that far more police activity and media interest is focused on the 'stranger danger' syndrome, than on the 'danger within'.

Does it feel less bad to be punched by a husband rather than a stranger, or is domestic violence so-called in order to suggest that such behaviour is almost to be expected within marriage? Is it an upsetting but understandable part of the relationship between partners? As such, it follows that it must be distinguished from the brutal random type of violence that peppers television programmes like *Crimewatch*. We need to reflect on the naming of the problem before we can attempt to consider possible reasons and possible solutions to such behaviour.

Domestic violence is generally considered to be an acceptable way of describing a pattern of physical and emotional assault that takes place in the home and is usually committed by males towards their adult partners. Largely replacing the well-known terms 'battered women' and 'battered wives', which focus on the victim rather than the assailant, it has come to be seen as a neutral catch-all term. Clearly the title 'battered wives', whilst perhaps drawing attention to the economically dependent position of many abused females, fails to suggest the wide range of relationships in which women are assaulted – not all women who are beaten are wives, some are mothers, daughters, lovers, and friends. More important, however, is the naming of the victim as the problem. What other crimes focus on the victim and then describe the victim as the problem?

Picture the following scenario: a middle-aged woman is run over and killed by a drunk driver. Would we refer to this as the problem of pedestrians? Similarly, would we refer to petty theft as the problem of market stalls? Only when we accurately name the problem as that of violent men instead of using a generalised term will we be able to start to discover why such violence occurs, whether it is rooted in the socialisation of boys or more fundamentally in the structure of society, which remains male dominated in all the major areas of power.

So why do midwives need to know and understand this aspect of our society? Midwives are in a unique position amongst health care workers. They are privileged to meet women at a very special, emotional and often deeply spiritual time in their lives. They meet women when they are about to undergo a major physical and psychological change in both their lives and in their role in society. For most women pregnancy is a major life event: it is the change from girl to woman and the passage from childhood to motherhood.

Midwives have the time and the opportunity to form a therapeutic relationship with childbearing women. We know from the research evidence that when midwives form this type of relationship with women during pregnancy, they are in a privileged position and have the opportunity to support, influence and stand alongside women as they undergo both physical and emotional change. Childbearing women often seek out the support of a kind, competent, caring health professional to guide them through the experience of childbirth. Many childbearing women will seek outside advice often for the first time; they will feel compelled, often for the sake of the unborn child, to seek professional help. If they meet an informed, caring, sensitive midwife, they are likely to lean heavily on her and place their trust in the relationship; it is not unusual for women, at this time of increased vulnerability, to share with another woman, perhaps for the first time, some previously secret aspects of their lives.

This openness, honesty, exposure of feelings and need for support represents an awesome responsibility for the listener. A well-informed midwife must understand the complexities of domestic violence; she needs to have the ability to respond appropriately and thus in some small way improve the woman's childbirth experience. The midwife can offer the support and guidance that may be needed not only for the months of pregnancy but also for the years ahead.

We also know that many midwives when confronted with the issue of domestic violence will, almost instinctively, give the woman clear direct advice. They will often angrily insist that the woman must leave the man who has inflicted the violence. This initial response, which stems from both the caring role combined with the traditional use of professional power, may well be totally inappropriate.

This book will help the midwife to understand the nature of violence, its roots, its manifestation in pregnancy and something of what can be done. It will help to guard against well-meaning professionals who offer advice that is not only unachievable, unrealistic, but also insensitive and has the potential to create more pain. The aim of the book is to help midwives help women more. It aims to increase the midwife's understanding of a very complex aspect of society, so as to enable her to stand alongside the woman as she faces an impossible future, to value her, be her friend and her advocate.

The book is written from a feminist perspective without excuse or apology and recognises the importance to all women of raising their self-esteem and feelings of self-worth in a patriarchal society.

The book has eight chapters, most of which include brief case studies and scenarios to illustrate the complexity of care and help apply theory to clinical midwifery practice. It draws on published research evidence, political and social comment and literature reviews wherever possible.

Chapter 1 explores domestic violence and sets the scene for the rest of the book. Chapter 2, which examines the shape of society, is important in assisting the reader to explore the causes of violence, which are discussed later in the book. Chapter 3 explodes the myths and stereotypes that surround domestic violence – many people believe that violence is a problem of the poor, the alcoholic and the black African. In Chapter 4 we peel back the layers of the onion and explore the causes of violence in a so-called civilised society.

Chapter 5 focuses on domestic violence and childbirth and sets out the extent and severity of domestic violence in pregnancy.

Chapter 6 focuses on the specific nursing and midwifery interventions open to clinicians. By exploring the complexities of power, the concepts of autonomy and the ability of the professionals to disempower abused women, this chapter challenges midwives and others to examine their role and contribution to the problem.

Chapter 7 – 'Who else can help?' – explores other options open to abused women. It considers and debates the statutory and voluntary provision, as well as the legal framework, to support women.

Finally, in Chapter 8 a summary and some conclusions are offered.

This book draws unashamedly on feminist insights: we believe that domestic violence is morally and socially outrageous and demands a distinct and radical response. The role of feminism in any consideration of social relationships may be thought by some to be old-fashioned and even irrelevant, given that for many, the term 'woman' has ceased to have any specific meaning. Post-structuralists, for example, suggest that the notion of any fixed category is problematic; that both women and men can be regarded as genderless beings, for whom there is no homogenous experience; no single voice which unites either sex. Instead, there are shifting and contradictory dimensions of identity which undermine the unifying 'truth' of shared experiences. Historically, feminist theories have been seen to provide competing explanations of women's oppression.

While such a structural, deterministic view of the social and cultural position of women may feel uncomfortable, especially for younger women brought up in a more liberal society, the fact remains that violence against women still exists, and is in fact commonplace. The feminist perspective itself encompasses a diversity of thought and a range of analyses, but fundamental to all feminisms is the simple yet radical aim to free women, not *from* oppression but *to* control their own lives without fear.

Clearly, not all men are bad; not all women are abused. Our book seeks to draw on the experiences of a few women to demonstrate the varied experiences of domestic violence, and the individualised responses to it. Their situations are all different and yet common themes emerge.

We have drawn on much of the available literature and have sought to identify these common threads, to indicate where similarities in experience suggest that the problem of violence against women is 'our' problem, not 'theirs'; an issue for society rather than the individual.

The role of agency in influencing the actions of both women and men cannot be overlooked in a post-modern society in which there are no universal truths; but we still need to be clear that for many women violence is a daily fact of life, for which they can never be held to blame.

We have avoided prescribing universal solutions but have urged midwives and others to look on women as individuals and support them as they seek the right pathway for themselves. We do not offer answers, but an opportunity to increase understanding and knowledge in this area.

Chapter 1

Exploring domestic violence and setting the scene

Yes he does knock me about a bit. It's mainly when he's drunk. I had a miscarriage once after I fell, well you know, sort of fell down the stairs. He felt really bad about that. He went back to his mother for a bit, but when he came back he was really great for a bit. He kept getting me things, you know jewellery and that.

In this chapter, we begin by exploring the definitions of domestic violence, and unpacking it as a concept. We look at the published data on prevalence and the costs to the public sector of domestic violence. We consider the history and ask 'who is beaten and who does the beating?' We begin to explore the literature relating to violence and the pregnant woman and the effects of violence on the unborn child. We explore the characteristics of battered women, searching for similarities and common themes. We use individuals' stories to illustrate the diversity of women's experiences.

What is domestic violence?

The 1993 Home Affairs Select Committee Report on domestic violence defined domestic violence as 'any form of physical, sexual or emotional abuse which takes place within the context of a close relationship. In most cases the relationship will be between partners who are married, cohabiting or otherwise, or ex-partners'. However, in this book we will try to look beyond such definitions.

The term domestic violence may conjure up a wealth of different images, but possibly the most common is that of the long-suffering wife with a black eye who has 'walked into a door'. Such images allow us to acknowledge the existence of domestic violence, but often prevent us from really appreciating the full extent and horror of such a practice. We may sympathise with this woman: we may believe that her husband is a bully, or that he has a quick temper or a drink problem; we may even think that whilst not justified, she had somehow brought the violence on herself, through her nagging, and so on. For some readers this will strike a chord, but for most, they may feel fortunate that they are not in such a relationship. Most of us, however, rarely go beyond this subjective response to consider why such violence is allowed to continue in our civilised society. By focusing only on those women with their black eyes, we can compartmentalise the problem, reducing the significance of it to an individual woman's problem. In this book, we hope to peel back the layers of the domestic violence 'onion' to make visible the appalling physical and mental suffering which thousands of women are experiencing daily. Many of these women are pregnant, often as a result of coercion or even rape. As midwives, we will meet these women. We need to try to understand their lives; we need to know how to respond if they seek our help; most of all, we need to be outraged that such a tradition still prevails. Understanding the complex factors involved in domestic violence can only quicken its eradication.

One of the first problems is that of defining domestic violence. Physical violence and our tolerance of it, may itself be, at least in part, subjective. A slap may be regarded by some as a form of communication, and by others as an assault on their person. To be 'slapped' by a drunken partner may be seen as par for the course in a relationship that is deemed to be generally satisfactory, whilst others may regard the same incident as a completely unacceptable expression of physical power. Some women may interpret non-physical acts, such as shouting or arguing, as violent, because this engenders fear in them; very often it is threats of violence that are perceived as terrifying. Others may feel that 'true' violence is only that which results in some form of visible injury. Whatever the level and nature of the violence, what unifies the experience is that it takes place within a close relationship and it serves the purpose of confirming the power structure within that relationship.

The commonly accepted understanding of domestic violence is the use of some degree of physical force, and this form of abuse is the most commonly documented, possibly because it is the most visible evidence of an abusive relationship. Evidence from Dobash and Dobash (1979) suggests that wife or partner assault makes up 25% of all violent crime, and that is likely to be an underestimation. Such assaults may include slapping, pushing, hitting with or throwing household objects, punching, kicking, the use of weapons and attempts to smother or strangle. Bourlet (1990) discovered a similar range of physical attacks in his research:

- Subject 105 was six months pregnant when she was run over deliberately by her husband in his lorry after an argument. She miscarried and lost the child.

- Subject 106 had been out to visit a friend, which annoyed her husband. He beat her with his fists, causing her a broken nose, black eyes and deadened facial nerves.

- Subject 107's husband started an argument at home. He beat her with his fists and feet, causing her two black eyes, a swollen nose and face, loss of some hair, a foot mark on the face and a cut finger.

– Following an argument over another woman, the husband of subject 108 assaulted her with his fists and feet, causing her broken ribs, black eyes and bruising all over.

Research on Scottish women in prison found examples of attacks including severe beatings, with physical injuries ranging from the loss of teeth and an eye, through to physical mutilation – a carved swastika on a woman's forehead. Examples of non-violent abuse are less well documented, often because it goes unseen for much longer, and because the effect of it can be even more terrifying than physical injuries. Many women experience sheer fear through verbal threats and taunts, but because there is no actual physical harm, they may be more affected by feelings of guilt, shame and so on – the feeling that they are somehow to blame, or that they shouldn't make a fuss. One such case is that of an author's wife who was tormented for many years with her inferiority, her lack of any social status independent of her husband, her uselessness as a wife and mother, and her totally meaningless existence. Her story is typical of so many others. This woman almost came to believe what she was told, and it was partly this false perception of herself that prevented her from leaving before she did. If she was completely worthless, she reasoned, perhaps she had the life she deserved?

The prevalence of domestic violence

In 1971, Dobash and Dobash (1980:2) observed that 'almost no-one had heard of battered women, except of course the legions of women who were being battered and the relatives, friends, ministers, social workers, doctors and lawyers in whom some of them confided.'

Over 12,000 women a year (Lovenduski and Randall, 1993:309) go to a refuge, and many thousands more experience violence but either seek alternative help or remain in the situation. Data gathered by Bakowski *et al.* (1983) suggests that women are likely to be subjected to violence in one in four marriages. Research from the United States suggests that between two and four million, and possibly as many as eight million women, are battered every year by the men they live with (Sassetti, 1993). Twenty-five per cent of all violent assaults in Britain are carried out on women by their partners (Lovenduski and Randall, 1993) and one in five British murder victims is a woman murdered by her partner or ex-partner (Smith, 1989).

In contrast, violence against men by their partners seems to account for just 1 per cent of reported violence, and there is some indication that such violence may be in the form of self-defence (Bakowski *et al.*, 1983). As with documented statistics about violence against women, the numbers of men reporting such incidences may be unrepresentative of the actual numbers experiencing such violence. However, notwithstanding the issue of under-reporting, female violence against men receives a disproportionate amount of media attention and appears to stimulate much more reaction than the infinitely more common abuse against women.

The most interesting fact about domestic violence statistics is that they are almost impossible to find. Most studies suggest that between one in three and one in four women report having suffered domestic violence at some time in their adult lives (Radford, Hester and Pearson, 1998). Most writers and the Home Office believe that the statistics are under-stated and as a crime domestic violence is under-reported. The Home Office collects details of the types of offences that are committed each year, but not the relationship of the offender to the victim unless the offence results in death. In 1996 the Criminal Statistics for England and Wales show that of 217 female homicide victims, 43 per cent were killed by their partners (defined as present or former spouse, co-habitant or lover), but of the 410 male homicide victims, only 6 per cent were killed by their partners. For offences of violence against the person in 1990-94 where the victim was a woman, just under half took place at the home of the victim or suspect (Watson, 1996).

The Biennial British Crime Survey (BCS) asked a representative sample of 16,500 adults in England and Wales directly about their experiences of crime and whether or not it was reported to the police. This survey found that in 1995 the incidents of domestic violence on women were estimated at one million; in 1997 the estimates fell to 835,000 but both of these figures are likely to be under-estimates. The same survey found that 43 per cent of all violent crime experienced by women was domestic and the number of domestic assaults reported to the BCS interviewers rose by 79 per cent between 1981 and 1991. It is estimated that only 25 per cent of all domestic violence incidents are reported to the police.

In January 1999 the Home Office published a new research study, based on a self-completion questionnaire (*Home Office Research Study 191*).

This study formed part of the 1996 British Crime Survey and was designed to maximise the victim's willingness to report domestic assaults and threats. It is claimed to be the most reliable study of domestic violence in England and Wales, even though it relies on self-reporting with all the inaccuracies of such a process. According to this survey, 4.2 per cent of women and 4.2 per cent of men said they had been physically assaulted by a current or former partner in the last year, and 4.9 per cent of men and 5.9 per cent of women had experienced physical assault and/or frightening threats. Women were twice as likely as men to have been injured by a partner in the last year, and three times as likely to have suffered frightening threats. They were also more likely to have been assaulted three or more times. Women were far more likely to say they had experienced domestic assault at some time in their lives: 23 per cent of women and 15 per cent of men, aged 16 to 59, said they had been physically assaulted by a current or former partner at some time. At least 12 per cent of women and 5 per cent of men had been assaulted on three or more occasions. In this survey, young women aged 20 to 24 reported the highest levels of domestic violence; 28 per cent said that they had been assaulted by a partner at some time and 34 per cent had been threatened or assaulted. This study also reports on those at highest risk of physical assault: it appears this includes those aged between 16 and 24; separated from their spouse; living in council property; in poor health; and/or in financial difficulties. Amongst men, victims were likely to be aged 16 to 24; unemployed; co-habiting and, like women, more likely to be in financial difficulties.

This survey has also asked questions about the nature of the assaults and the assailants. It was found that pushing, shoving and grabbing were the most common types of assault but kicking, slapping and hitting with fists took place in nearly half of the reported incidences. Women were more likely to be injured and more likely to report that they had been frightened by the experience. The study defined those who had been assaulted on three or more occasions as 'chronic victims'. Such victims experienced more serious types of attack; they were more likely to be physically injured and were more emotionally affected by their experience. Three quarters of the chronic victims were women. The survey found that virtually all incidents against women were committed by men and 95 per cent of those against men were committed by women. The assailant was said to be under the influence of alcohol in 32 per cent of incidents and of drugs in 5 per cent. Only half of those assaulted had told someone about their most recent assault and only 12 per cent of incidents were reported to the police. Medical staff were told of only 10 per cent of incidents. It was clear from the study that victims believed that they were in some way responsible for the assault and this influenced the decision to report the experience. Only 17 per cent of victims thought that their experience was a crime. It could be argued that a relatively minor incident, such as a push or shove, might be remembered and reported by an individual, especially if such action was highly unusual or a one-off incident. For many women, the daily grind of physical and emotional abuse may lead them to consider the behaviour 'normal' and, as such, not worth reporting. Many critics of domestic violence statistics argue that minor injuries are a normal part of complex relationships. It is important to recognise that assault is a crime and should be recognised as such.

The authors of the BCS domestic violence report believe that the incidence may well be under-reported. They argue that as the questionnaire was part of the BCS it may have led respondents to believe the survey was only interested in crime. Many women may have become so used to violence that they do not see it as a crime. The report also recognises that interviewing women in their own homes might inhibit disclosure; this factor, combined with a natural reluctance to relive traumatic personal experiences, may well limit the disclosure. Respondents to a survey of this nature may also exaggerate incidents for effect. It is unlikely that these effects cancel each other out. The BCS concludes that domestic violence is a widespread problem with nearly one in four women assaulted by a partner at some time in their lives and one in eight repeatedly assaulted (1999:61).

Other studies

Radford, Hester and Pearson (1998) have produced a domestic violence fact sheet for the Women's Aid Federation, which brings together many of the published studies on the UK incidence of domestic violence, some of which are included here. Andrews and Brown's (1988) ten-year-old survey of marital violence in Islington found that 25 per cent of women with children had been subjected to violence by their partner. Dominy and Radford (1996) report the findings of a survey of 484 women in

Surrey's shopping centres. Here they found that one in four women defined themselves as having suffered domestic violence from a male partner, or ex-partner, since the age of 18 years. Two out of three women who defined themselves as victims of domestic violence had not told their family, friends or agencies about the abuse.

In another study, McGibbon, Cooper and Kelly (1988) found that out of 281 women attending GP surgeries in West London one in three reported suffering abuse from a male partner.

In a more recent study of 129 women attending GP surgeries, Stanko, Crisp, Hale and Lucraft (1997) found that one in nine reported experiences of domestic violence serious enough to require medical attention in the past twelve months.

In Islington in 1993, a survey of 430 women indicated that up to one-third of women are regularly physically or emotionally abused and one in three women had experienced domestic violence at some time in their lives, and twelve per cent had been victims of domestic violence in the previous year (Mooney, 1993). In Canada, a telephone survey of 11,000 women found that one in three women reported violence from their partners (Statistics Canada, 1996). Painter (1991) in a survey conducted in city centres in North England found that one in eight women reported having been raped by their husbands or partners.

The Women's Aid Federation publishes an annual survey of refuges. In the 1996/97 survey it was found that:

- At least 54,500 women and children spent at least one night in a refuge. Of this figure, approximately 32,017 were children and 22,492 were women.

- 145,315 women experiencing domestic violence called refuges and support services.

- 67,192 of these calls were from women seeking refuge and 69,875 calls were from women requesting advice and support.

- The largest group (41 per cent) of women using refuge services were aged between 26 and 35 years. Nearly 25 per cent were aged between

19 and 25 years and 20 per cent between 36 and 45 years.

– On leaving refuge accommodation, 29 per cent were successfully re-housed in either local authority or housing association properties and only 6 per cent went into private rented accommodation. Nearly 10 per cent went to stay with friends and relatives and 15 per cent moved onto another refuge. Just over 12 per cent returned home with an injunction against their violent partner, and nearly 20 per cent returned to their abuser.

Costs to the public sector of domestic violence

The financial costs of domestic violence, as opposed to the physical, emotional and psychological costs, are only just beginning to be considered. In a new report by Stanko *et al.* (1998), published by Crime Concern, the researchers estimated in 1996 the total cost to the public sector of providing services for women and children facing domestic violence in Hackney to be around £90 per annum per household. They also estimated the total cost for Greater London to be around £278 million per annum. This considerable drain on resources may act as a trigger to a more significant Government response to violence. In that study 10 per cent of women surveyed reported being knocked unconscious by their partners and 5 per cent had sustained broken bones.

The history of domestic violence

Domestic violence is not a twentieth century phenomenon, any more than generalised violence could be said to be a modern 'disease'. Undoubtedly, it has existed as long as close relationships between women and men have existed – thousands of years. There is evidence of its presence in Roman times; indeed the popular children's figure Mr Punch is derived from a Roman mime called 'Maccus' (Brewer, 1978). (The idea that a puppet show depicting a violent husband could be suitable entertainment for our young children will be followed up later.)

The Bible – the foundation of all Judeo-Christian beliefs – tells the story of the first couple, Adam and Eve. It is a tale of seduction, disobedience, weakness, all committed by the female, and has in many ways formed the basis of the common expectations of how women are and are not supposed to behave. Indeed, until relatively recently, a woman was expected to obey her husband upon marriage, a concept which clearly implies the right of the husband to some form of control and correction if not adhered to. Similarly, the religion of Judaism has been followed for several thousand years: its (male) supporters have long been using the following prayer response in the morning service:

> *Blessed art thou, O Lord our God, King of the Universe, who hast not made me a woman.* (The Jewish Book of Prayer)

That some of the traditional ideology of male dominance remains within that culture can be seen by the fact that there are women's refuges in contemporary Israel (Dobash and Dobash, 1979).

The link between religion and wife-beating has long been established. The 'sanctity of marriage' (a sacrament of course) has been and still is used to account for such behaviour, and to suggest reasons why women should continue to endure it. The institution of marriage is often regarded as paramount to all other situations, as evidenced by the following account given by Linda, an American woman:

> *Mom. Chuck has beaten me bloody ... He has held a gun to my head and made me do awful things. He has forced me to have sex with women and other men. And now he is talking about making me have sex with animals. He is turning me into a prostitute. He is always threatening to kill me. He has even threatened to kill you and Daddy ...*
>
> *But Linda, he's your 'husband'.* (Stanko, 1992).

Far-fetched? Very probably, but nonetheless a true account (not disputed) given by a witness in a prosecution case against her husband.

Simone de Beauvoir (translated in 1974) highlighted the link between Christianity and the law:

> *Man enjoys the great advantage of having a god endorse the code*

he writes; and since man exercises a sovereign authority over women, it is especially fortunate that this authority has been vested in him by the Supreme Being.

In other words, if God gives powerful authority to men to exercise as they see fit, if they choose to use such authority against women in whatever form, then God can be seen to justify wife-beating.

Evidence of domestic violence has also come to light from the civilisations of Ancient Egypt, where it is said that a woman who spoke out against her husband was liable to having her teeth hit with a brick (Bourlet, 1990).

The tradition of accepting domestic violence goes back much further than the tradition of deploring it. Indeed, until the nineteenth century British husbands had a legal right to beat their wives for what was considered to be 'lawful correction'. The legal situation has been summarised by Blackstone (1765/cited by Bourlet, 1990) as follows:

The husband also might give his wife moderate correction. For as he is to answer for her misbehaviour, the law thought it reasonable to entrust him with this power of restraining her, 'by domestic chastisement in the same moderation that a man is allowed to correct his servant or his children'. A general 'rule of thumb' operated in the courts, whereby husbands were not permitted to use a stick broader than a thumb, but not after 10pm or at the weekends, as this might disturb the neighbours praying.

It is significant that legal reform in the guise of the Matrimonial Causes Act 1878, followed after the Cruelty to Animals Act 1876, which extended the scope of the previous Cruelty to Animals Act of 1849. This latter Act had made it illegal to 'cruelly beat, ill-treat, over-drive, abuse or torture' any domestic animal. Clearly, dogs and cats had better protection in their own homes than did women.

We will be discussing the current legal position in Chapter 7, but the evidence suggests that the culture of accepting domestic violence remains, irrespective of changes in the law.

Who is beaten?

The highest reported incidence of domestic violence is among lower socio-economic groups – the poor. However, much qualitative research suggests that such crime is experienced by women of all classes, ages and ethnic background (Radford, 1987; Kelly *et al.*, 1991). A random survey conducted by Mooney (1993) discovered that 30 per cent of women had experienced violence (more severe than being pushed or shaken) by a current or former partner. In addition, 23 per cent had been raped, 27 per cent had been threatened and 37 per cent had been subjected to mental cruelty. Negligible differences were found relating to class or ethnicity.

Differences in the actual rate of reporting may be accounted for by the fact that poorer women may have no alternative but to seek help from the police, refuges, hospitals, and so on. Middle-class women may have a network of supportive family and friends who can provide shelter and support, undermining the need to go to the police. This group may also be more traumatised into silence, as so much less is known about the incidence of domestic violence amongst them. A truly vicious circle.

Wife-beating occurs throughout the whole world: Germany (Hagemann White, 1981), Israel (Saunders, 1982), the Mediterranean (Loizos, 1978), Amazonia (Chagnon, 1968), and Mexico (Roldan, 1982). Schlegel rated forty-five societies and showed that three-quarters of them permitted husbands to be aggressive to their wives (Schlegel, 1972).

Both victims and their attackers may be young or old; for example, a woman of 82 sought refuge accommodation after years of abuse by her now dead husband. Following a brief respite, her son had taken up his father's 'role' and the woman was forced to leave the house where she had lived for over fifty years. In short, the rich, the poor, the able bodied, the disabled, celebrities, superstars, athletes, the unemployed – all may beat or be beaten. Domestic violence occurs in every dimension of society, but most of the time if it isn't happening to us we can't recognise it.

Who does the beating?

Both men and women can be violent, and indeed the Campaign against Family Violence recommends that physicians be encouraged to identify male victims of abuse as well as female victims. However, recent statistics from the USA suggest that 95 per cent of domestic violence victims are female (US Department of Justice statistics), and that in terms of violent conduct by both sexes, it is men who use more dangerous and injurious forms of violence, do more damage due to their physical strength, use repeated violence (Strauss *et al.*, 1980) and even when unarmed, pose more of a physical menace to women than vice versa (Browne, 1993).

It is also important to recognise the different motivations behind violence: men may attack their partners because something was not done in the 'right' manner; or because they have not got their own way; or to show they are in charge. Women's use of violence is much more likely to be in self-defence of either an ongoing or threatened attack, or as a moment of anger after possibly years of abuse, usually perpetrated when their partner is vulnerable – either asleep or drunk. This latter context is now being hotly debated in legal circles; it has not been recognised as self-defence if there was no violent behaviour by the partner in evidence at the time. However, many women have argued that they would not have dared to retaliate against their partners if fully awake, and that such action is a form of self-defence against certain future abuse.

In a society in which women are gaining some power, it may well be that female aggression becomes more commonplace, but it is also likely that such behaviour will be focused towards other females – at school, amongst peer groups and so on, and not directed at partners with whom there is likely to remain an unequal relationship, partly due to the continued economic dependence of many women on their partners. Dublin Women's Aid have drawn up a list of 'Don'ts' for women in violent relationships, which suggest that far from women becoming equal in relationships, they must actually still subjugate their own wishes to those of their partners, often to an extreme extent. This list is shown in Figure 1.1.

The message from these guidelines is quite simply that in many cases violence is inevitable; it is often completely unrelated to the behaviour of the abused woman, if that could indeed be used to justify a violent response, and must leave all of us with the guiding principle, espoused by many Zero Tolerance campaigns – 'There is never an excuse'.

- Don't wear make-up. If you do he'll call you a slut.
- Don't not wear make-up. He'll call you a slob.
- Don't ask your friend round. He won't want the house full of chattering females.
- Don't not ask your friend round. Are you ashamed of him or something?
- Don't have dinner on the table when he gets in. He'll think you are getting at him for being late.
- Don't let dinner be late. The least a man deserves when he gets in after a long day is to have his dinner ready on the table.
- Don't let the children get in his way. He'll be too tired to bother with a lot of screaming kids.
- Don't send them to bed before he gets home. Do you want them to forget their father?
- Don't ask him what kind of day he's had. You should be able to see just by looking at him that it's been dreadful.
- Don't forget to ask how his day was. A woman should show some interest in what a man's doing.
- Don't tell him about your day. He doesn't want to hear a lot of complaints.
- Don't not tell him about your day. Are you hiding something from him?
- Don't put on a sexy negligee at bedtime. You look like a whore, and anyway, whose money do you think you are spending?
- Don't go to bed in your pyjamas. A man needs something attractive to sleep with occasionally.
- Don't put your arms around him in bed. When he wants it, he'll ask for it.
- Don't turn over and go to sleep. Are you frigid or what?
- And lastly:
- Don't fight back when he hits you. It might make him worse.
- Don't whatever you do, don't be scared. It'll make him feel guilty, so he'll hit you more.
- Follow these few little tips and you'll never be battered again. Unless of course you ask for it ...

(Women's Aid, Dublin 1993)

Figure 1.1 Don'ts for women in violent relationships

Violence and the pregnant woman

This topic will be explored in more detail in Chapter 5. Women living in ongoing abusive relationships are more likely to be battered once they become pregnant (Helton *et al.*, 1987; Strauss *et al.*, 1980). Studies have shown that 40-60 per cent of previous domestic violence victims are beaten while pregnant (McFarlane *et al.*, 1992). However, very often, a woman's announcement of her pregnancy leads directly to an assault by her partner. In fact, pregnancy may be a trigger factor of the very first assault, leading to a relationship of beatings. Violence towards pregnant women has been referred to as child abuse in the womb, undeniably accurate, but perhaps a way of suggesting that violence against all women is less important unless they are pregnant? That there can be no justification at all for hitting a pregnant woman, no way in which she could have deserved it, which seems to suggest that it is possible that non-pregnant women may be to blame for their own abuse in some way.

Pregnant women may display a wide variety of injuries and complaints; some may seek treatment, others may not. The usual gory list of injuries have been reported by women who are pregnant, but there often appears to be a different pattern of injury inflicted by partners. The abdomen appears to be the commonest site, followed by other parts of the body usually hidden from public view, such as the ribs and buttocks (Stewart and Cecutti, 1993). This may signify some awareness of guilt about such actions, and the possible social disapproval they would engender. Or it may simply be a desire to keep such activities secret in order that they may be carried on indefinitely.

Thelma's story is typical of so many (see Figure 1.2).

Thelma's story

Following an incident at a relative's party at which her husband accused Thelma of flirting with another man, 'I tried to reassure myself that he wouldn't hit me when I was so heavily pregnant (6 months). I was wrong. When we reached the house he dragged me out of the car by my hair. I pleaded with him not to hurt the baby. He reminded me that I had an appointment at the antenatal clinic the following morning, and that instead of beating me he was going to punish me. He made me sit at the kitchen table with my hand placed flat out. He went to the garage, returning with a hammer. He asked me which two fingers I wanted broken. I had ten seconds to answer. I tried to reason with him, but without warning he smashed the hammer down onto the last two fingers of my left hand ... He made me sit at that table all night. I had to urinate in the chair. In the morning, he told me to clean myself up and get ready for the clinic ... I couldn't tell the doctor what had happened, although he was visibly shocked at the state of my hand. He asked me if everything was all right at home. I told him it was. I desperately did want everything to be all right. I was also too frightened of what would happen if I did tell anyone.

Brian left me alone after that night. The next beating wasn't until the baby was 15 weeks old. I had been up most of the night and had overslept in the morning. I hadn't got his breakfast ready. He threw eggs and bacon at me and then said he was going to pour petrol over me – that way he would know his breakfast was cooking. The beatings became a regular occurrence after that time and especially after the birth of our second child. During my third pregnancy, Brian kicked me and threw me downstairs – I lost that baby. In my next pregnancy, every hour was spent avoiding conflict. I even slept with one leg out of the bed, as I felt I would be able to escape more easily if he woke up in a rage. Three weeks before the baby was due, I was admitted to hospital with high blood pressure. I stayed in until the birth. I could sleep at night, I was relaxed, and most of all my baby was safe . My other children were staying with a neighbour and seeing it as a bit of an adventure. Brian only came in once a week. I still look back on that time when my little boy was born, I couldn't stop crying. People thought I was happy, but it was because I didn't want to go home. I just prayed and prayed that Brian would have a heart attack or a car accident. The beatings started again when the baby was two weeks old.

Figure 1.2 Thelma's story

Violence and the unborn child

This issue is explored in more detail in Chapter 5. The most obvious and serious risk to the unborn child is that of death. Injury to the mother's abdomen, such as being punched or kicked, can cause fetal death by placental separation or abruption. Reliable statistics are hard to come by due to the fairly common situation of naturally occurring spontaneous abortions, and the desire by many abused women to maintain secrecy about the possible causes of their miscarriages. However, research suggests that women who are battered are four times more likely to have miscarriages than those who are not (Bullock and McFarlane, 1989). Assaults can also cause such injuries as fetal fractures, brain damage and rupture of internal organs. Apart from these direct effects of violence, babies of battered women are more likely to have a low birth weight. This may reflect the higher rate of smoking, drinking and the use of medication and illicit drugs, which many abused women turn to as a means of coping (Amaro *et al.*, 1990). Such women often believe that the survival of their unborn baby is due to chance and is therefore outside their control. However they treat their bodies it cannot guarantee the safe delivery of a healthy baby (Stewart and Cecutti, 1993). However, low birth weight is seen as a reliable predictor of infant wellness and future development.

Characteristics of battered women

It has already been seen that women who are battered come from all backgrounds and lifestyles, but do they have anything in common? Is it possible to identify any qualities in their personalities which may make it more likely that they will end up in an abusive relationship? In her study, Walker (1984) identified nine common characteristics of women who had been battered. A victim of domestic violence commonly:

- Had low self-esteem and felt inadequate about her abilities.

- Believed all of the myths about battering relationships; for example, as a woman she had somehow caused the violence.

- Believed in the traditional roles of men and women in the home and viewed the man as the head of the household and felt that she was incapable of taking care of herself and had to be dependent on a man.

- Believed that she could keep the batterer from becoming angry and accepted responsibility for the batterer's actions. In so doing she could avoid future violence.

– Suffered from guilt but denied the terror and anger she felt.

– Presented a passive face to the world but had the strength to manipulate her environment enough to prevent further violence and being killed.

– Had severe stress reactions with psychological and physiological complaints.

– Used sex as a way to establish intimacy, in the hope of making violence less likely.

– Believed that no one would be able to help her resolve her predicament but herself.

Boyd and Klingbeil (1993) in Schornstein (1997) identified twenty-one common characteristics of domestic violence victims. In addition to the above, they also found that an abused woman commonly:

– Was both economically and emotionally dependent, and was often using large quantities of drugs and alcohol secretly.

– Was unsure of her own ego needs and defined herself in terms of partner, children, family, job and other external components.

– Had an unrealistic hope that change was imminent and believed in 'promises' that things would get better.

– Experienced gradually increasing social isolation, including loss of contact with immediate family and friends.

– Had a generational history of witnessing abuse in her family.

– Participated in 'pecking order' abuse; sometimes she would treat those of lower status, such as her children, in an abusive way.

– Was at high risk for assault and other abuse during pregnancy.

– Frequently contemplated suicide and had a history of minor attempts and frequently wished that her partner was dead.

– Experienced an inability to convince her partner of her loyalty.

Many of these characteristics are demonstrated by Carole, a young woman of 16 (see Figure 1.3).

Carole's story

Carole had experienced a troubled childhood. Her father had constantly beaten her mother in front of her, and she had stayed in refuges with her mother and brother on numerous occasions. Her relationship with her mother eventually broke down and she went into care. She left at 16, drifted in and out of bedsits and then met Steve, a 31-year-old plumber. He had a good job, and was generous with his money. He really seemed to care for her. After a few weeks, Steve asked Carole to move in with him, and she was thrilled.

On their first evening, Steve returned from work to discover that Carole had cleaned up, moving some of his possessions. He was furious and Carole was very frightened, although he didn't hit her then. Over the following weeks, Carole became more and more confused as Steve would change from being sweet and kind one moment to terrifying her the next. He started asking her how she had spent her day, accusing her of seeing other men. He began ringing her several times a day to check on her whereabouts. On one occasion, he accused her of lying about going shopping, because he believed she had been much longer than necessary. Despite her protestations, he beat her, then went out. On his return he was very apologetic, telling Carole that he was frightened of her leaving him. Carole tried to convince him that she would never do so, and that she would try harder to please him. Several weeks passed without incident and Carole began to relax. Then one day, Steve brought a large dog home, despite knowing that Carole was frightened of them. He told her that the dog was to guard her, and prevent her from seeing other men. Every morning he would leave the dog in the hall. Carole was too frightened to go out through the front door (the only exit). On his return from work, Steve would often take her shopping, and was nice to her. Confused again, Carole would often try to plead with Steve to let her go out. One such episode ended with Steve violently assaulting her, knocking one of her teeth out.

Again, Carole agreed she would try to behave 'better'. Two days later, Steve arrived with flowers and a small present. It was her tooth, mounted on a gold chain. He hung it around her neck. When she started to cry, he beat her, kicking her in the stomach several times. The neighbours next door heard her screams, louder than usual, and called the police. She was taken to hospital, where she had a miscarriage. She gave Steve as her next of kin.

> She denied that she had been beaten and left hospital a few days later with Steve. The relationship continued until Carole bumped into her mother whilst out with Steve. After several clandestine visits from her mother, she agreed to leave the flat, and was helped to move to another town. She refused to go to the police because she believed that deep down Steve did love her and needed help.

Figure 1.3 Carole's story

Further evidence that women often blame themselves for the eruption of violence can be seen in the example of Caroline Scott, the wife of the actor Shaun Scott. The story was reported in the *Daily Mail*, 7 January 1998:

> *I honestly believe it's my fault ... when I look where he's hit me, I feel like I deserve it. I know I've failed.*

Such expressions of guilt are all too familiar, and reflect the way in which it is the abusers who define the reality of the situation, by suggesting that they have been driven to violence by the behaviour of their partners.

Research has also been focused on the batterers, and appears to suggest that they, too, may exhibit common characteristics. Walker (1984) found that they frequently:

- Had low self-esteem and felt inadequate.

- Believed all of the myths about battering relationships, including the belief that women provoked violence by their behaviour

- Were traditionalists, believing in the stereotyped male sex role within the family, that is that the man should be the head of the household.

- Many, as children, had witnessed their father beat their mother or were beaten themselves.

- Blamed others for their actions.

- Tended to be irrationally jealous.

- Presented a dual personality, that is they appeared caring and loving to others whilst abusing their partner at home.

- Experienced high levels of stress; they used drinking and violence to help them to cope.

- Frequently used sex as an act of aggression to enhance self-esteem.

- Did not believe that their violent behaviour should have negative consequences or was a major problem in their relationships.

Again, Boyd and Klingbeil (1993) identified even more common aspects of identity. They found that abusive men often:

- Had an explosive and unpredictable temper and could not control their impulses.

- Were emotionally dependent and subject to deep depressions known only to their families.

- Had insatiable ego needs and displayed a quality of childlike narcissism that was not generally detectable to those outside the family. They made constantly exaggerated claims about their own abilities.

- Lacked guilt or remorse on an emotional level even after an intellectual recognition.

- Became increasingly more dangerous and posed more of a threat to family members over time.

- Perceived themselves as having poor social skills, describing their relationship with their partners as the closest they had known.

- Contained and/or confined their partners and employed devious tactics against them (for example, checked mileage and timed errands).

- Became increasingly violent when their partners were pregnant, with pregnancy often marking the first assault.

- Exerted control over their partners by threatening murder or suicide, often attempted one or both when their partners tried to leave them, and were known to actually complete either or both.

– Frequently used the children as 'pawns', exerted power and control through custody issues, and might have kidnapped or held the children hostage.

It appears that both the battered and the batterers have some characteristics in common: low self-esteem, belief in the traditional roles of men and women, and have often experienced or seen violence in their childhood.

Such shared characteristics may make it easier to view both parties as victims, although of course one group has much more power than the other. It is important to refrain from blaming the partners of abused women. It is not the role of midwives to stand in judgement, not least because this may well alienate the pregnant woman and make it less likely that she will be able to receive any help or support that she may need.

Perhaps the suggested characteristics of many batterers also allow us to go some way to understanding how pregnancy can be a flashpoint for violence. Men who are emotionally dependent on their partners may experience uncontrollable jealousy when asked to share their mate with another. In a sense they are 'acting out' the child within themselves (Berne, 1968) seeking unconditional and unlimited love; when this appears to be (in their eyes) reduced their response is fear and anger, which in turn becomes violence.

A fuller understanding of the complexities surrounding domestic violence is essential if midwives are to reach one of the most vulnerable groups of pregnant women – and a broader understanding will also help women (and men) in general. Domestic violence is *our* problem, not 'hers', 'his' or 'theirs'. Only when we all acknowledge that all women and children are potentially at risk, can we begin to change the nature of society that allows it to continue.

This chapter has clarified some of the terms and concepts that we use in the book. We have begun to set the scene for the story that follows. In the next chapter we will explore the shape of society and consider the impact of society on the issue of violence.

Chapter 2

The shape of society

I can't stand it when he gets angry. You know he gets sort of sexed up; then I know there will be trouble. He knocked my tooth out.

Yes, he has knocked me about. I have thought of leaving him, but this house is in my name. It no good calling the police round 'ere. They say it's a domestic and unless someone is getting hurt, they won't come. See, he can't understand why I've gone off it since I've been pregnant. It makes no difference, he just does it anyway.

I think he will go and stay with his other girlfriend when the baby is born.

In this chapter, we will be looking at what could be called the trigger factors to domestic violence. Do males, both boys and adults, appear to use violence more frequently than females? If so, is this because of biological differences or sociological influences? Are girls naturally more caring, or do we really want 'boys to be boys' in spite of talk about them needing to become more sensitive and emotional? Is violence an individual response, or are violent adults ' not born but made' by society?

Sex and gender

One of the commonest utterances of a midwife must surely be 'Congratulations! It's a boy!' or 'Well Done! You've got a *little* girl!' In that first moment of life we are identified as one sex or the other, based on our obvious physical differences. The common-sense emphasis on anatomical differences often leads to assumptions about intellectual and emotional differences between males and females. In this chapter we will seek to question whether biological differences are really significant enough to account for the vast differences in the way males and females are perceived – from what skills are attributed to each sex, to the differing choice of leisure activities. Although it is no longer widely believed that men are intellectually superior to women, it is still the prevailing view that males are drawn to particular subjects like maths, science and technology, whilst females naturally gravitate towards 'softer' subjects such as English, languages, and the humanity subjects. These patterns can be observed in the national A-level results, which Sears (1992) has concluded show no signs of any change in the number of girls taking science A levels despite the introduction of the National Curriculum. Of course, such statistics really only show how successful has been the process of creating preferences and aptitudes based on sex, rather than evidence for the existence of intellectual ability linked to different biological genitalia.

The term 'sex' then, can be used to refer to physical characteristics that differentiate females from males. Many such differences are obvious; apart from the sex organs, there is also a completely different reproductive system. Women alone are able to bear and suckle babies and it is this exclusively female ability that appears to be at the heart of ideas about the different natures of women and men. Since women grow infants it is often assumed that they must also be responsible for childcare, and most of the domestic duties associated with homemaking. The idea of sex (i.e. physical characteristics) determining the roles we play leads to the necessary distinction between sex and gender roles. Our sex role relates to whether we are male or female; whether we will determine the sex of children or whether we will actually provide nourishment for growing fetuses in utero. Our gender role, however, implies a way of feeling and behaving which is expected of us, according to our biology. We are expected to behave in either a masculine or a feminine way, as determined by our chromosomal origins. Girls are caring, kind, painstaking (passive); boys are boisterous, physical, adventurous (active). How much of our masculine or feminine behaviour is due to the pervasive conditioning of our society rather than any hormonal or genetic influence?

This distinction between the two concepts of sex and gender is, however, more ambiguous than at first appears. Whilst implying that gender is shaped by social factors (environment, and so on), it also implies that there are two distinct biological sexes. Many writers now believe that while there are differences between men and women, these are massively exaggerated.

Birke (1992) stresses that scientific work on sex differences looks at an average picture within the population, but there are many who deviate from these averages: women who are strong, tall, physically active ; men who are short, of slight build, non-aggressive, sedentary. According to Birke, biological and cultural factors should be viewed as 'interacting factors' – what is important is how humans culturally interpret biology and how the biological is shaped by the social.

Supporters of the biological determinist view argue that male traits are rooted in chromosomal differences (for example, XYY chromosomes) or in hormonal differences (for example, testosterone) or in some other natural characteristic that distinguishes women from men. If this were true, we would surely expect universal differences between the two, throughout the world. No such evidence is forthcoming however; indeed, several anthropological studies appear to contradict such an idea. In her study *Sex and Temperament in Three Primitive Societies*, Margaret Mead (1935) describes three tribes living in New Guinea: the Tchambuli, the Mundugumor and the Arapesh. The Tchambuli recognise a clear difference between the sexes; males are very definitely allotted distinct gendered characteristics, as are females. What is surprising however, is that males showed what we would call 'female' characteristics and the females displayed 'masculine' qualities. The men wear lovely ornaments, do the shopping, carve and paint and dance. The women are self-assertive, practical and manage all the affairs of the household.

Among the Arapesh, the ideal adult is passive, gentle and nurturing (what we might call feminine virtues) and no distinction at all is made between the sexes. The main work of both men and women is child-bearing and child-rearing. Sexual intercourse is called 'work', where the goal is to achieve a pregnancy, and the verb 'to give birth' is used for both sexes. The opposite is true amongst the Mundugumor, where both sexes appear to follow our traditional male pattern. The women are as aggressive and forceful as the men; they hate bearing and rearing children, whilst the men detest pregnancy in their wives. Children are carried in harsh baskets that scratch their skin, well away from their mother's breast. Children are raised to be independent and hostile, just like the adults.

These examples seem to suggest that the behavioural differences that we often believe are natural and are related to our physiological make-up, are actually quite arbitrary, in that it is the society in which we live that determines how we believe males and females should behave. There appears to be no universal blueprint for say, male behaviour, which therefore must lead us to question how influential our biological differences actually are.

Are gender differences mainly socially constructed then? Much research would seem to suggest so. Some researchers took four babies, all 6 months old, and dressed them all half the time in boys' clothes and half the time in girls' clothes. The 'girls' wore pretty, frilly dresses and were called Jane; the 'boys' wore blue suits and were called John. Eight mothers, who all had first born babies of about the same age, were then invited to play with the babies for a short period of time. The results were illuminating. When they believed the babies to be boys, the mothers encouraged them to be physically active and adventurous and often gave them a hammer-shaped rattle. When the babies were thought to be girls, the mothers chose a pink doll for the baby to play with, cuddled them a lot, often appeared to discourage them being adventurous and frequently remarked how pretty the baby was. Similar findings were reported by Rubin *et al.* (1974), when the parents of fifteen newborn (0-24 hours old) girls and fifteen newborn boys were interviewed. Despite there being no noticeable differences between the height and weight of the babies, the girls were seen as being smaller, more delicate and less attentive than the boys. It appears that the common practice of placing either a pink or a blue identification band around a new born's wrist has far reaching consequences.

The psychology of gender

We have touched on the influence of socialisation in the formation of gendered identities, and we shall return to that discussion shortly. Firstly, however, it is important to consider the psychological theories that have been put forward to account for the observable differences in behaviour and attitudes between males and females. As the main focus of this book is domestic violence, it is appropriate to concentrate on the differences observable in the institution of the family, the site of such activity. Examination of the family provides much information about the typical behaviour of women and men, boys and girls, their psychological dispositions and the roles that are considered to be gender appropriate.

Although these days most psychologists would regard both nature and nurture as influential in the psychological development of children, it is the dynamics of development through time that forms the basis of the cognitive developmental view – the study of the progressive interaction between the child and the environment. Lawrence Kohlberg (1966) believed that the child was an active agent in its development of sex-typed behaviour. He proposed that once a child understood the concept of gender, she or he then behaves according to the appropriate gender role. In other words, once a child understands what it means to be a boy, he will do 'boy' things.

Kohlberg suggests that the concept of gender develops through the following three stages:

1. *Gender identity (from 2 years old).* By the time it is 2, a child knows what gender it is, and is able to identify the sex of someone else, based

on appearance, clothes and so on.

2. *Gender stability (from 4 years old)*. By this age children know that they will stay the same sex throughout life, and that this applies to everyone although they can be deceived by appearances (for example, if a man is wearing women's clothing).

3. *Gender constancy (about 6 years old)*. By this time children know that although the appearance of something changes, its essential qualities do not. Once the idea that gender is constant has developed, a child will use the appropriate behaviour and copy the appropriate role models. For example, the six-year-old boy, recognising that he is a boy, would select football for viewing on the television, knowing that this is a 'boy's' activity.

Kohlberg's view is that as children come to regard themselves as girls or boys, they become positive in their beliefs about their own gender and negative about the opposite one. This feature for preference of their own gender is seen to guide the process of imitation and reinforcement – from about the age of 5, children appear to pay more attention to same-sex models. It is difficult to isolate the reasons for such behaviour, however, as later research has shown that parents not only reinforce behaviour that they deem appropriate for the child's sex, but they also provide toys they see as appropriate – in Western cultures, dolls for girls, cars for boys, for example (Rheingold and Cook, 1975).

It can be seen that such a theory is in fact a circular one – children become aware of their own gender identity, partly through observing the behaviour of adults of their own gender, but who has influenced the behaviour of the adults? Although we have seen that gender differences do differ dramatically between cultures, nevertheless underlying trends are observable. In nearly all cultures, men are more likely to initiate sex than women, men are more aggressive than women, and so on. It is not good enough to suggest that sexual stereotypes are responsible for the roles we associate with gender. We also need to explain how such stereotypes have been formed and why they still retain some influence. Theories of evolution can be used to explore the existence of stereotypes, by relating them to the historical biological context of natural selection. This concept purports that it produces behaviour that will maximise the reproductive success of individuals. As males and females have different reproductive requirements, they have developed different predispositions to acquire particular types of behaviour (Hinde and Stevenson-Hinde, 1973). What are these differing behaviours? A male, to stand a chance of parenthood, must merely inseminate a female, whereas a female must nurture the embryo, fetus and infant through pregnancy and lactation. Competition is therefore greater between males for females than between females for males. Natural selection has operated to make males more competitive, and hence physically stronger and more aggressive than females. Also, since females always know that they are the mothers of their children, whereas males can never be completely sure, the process of natural selection has ensured that children are more important to the female than to the male – a clear indication of what appears to be a biological cause of the traditional division of labour in a family, and an obvious reason for maintaining such a structure.

Is male aggression natural?

Most violence, most crime ... is not committed by human beings in general. It is committed by men. (Tweedie, *The Guardian*, April 27, 1978)

Organisations that have powers of social control, such as the police or the army, and which may legally use force consist largely of men. Similarly, large crowds, such as football supporters, which may be considered as having the potential for violence, are again, mainly male. Violence is seen as the 'masculine way of reacting to the difficulties and frustrations of life' (Archer and Lloyd, 1989:124). Females, on the other hand, are expected to respond more passively. Does this mean that men are biologically programmed to be more aggressive, or is it merely more acceptable for males to display aggression, although females experience the emotion equally? How is the concept of aggression defined in this context – do minor acts of violence, verbal abuse or losing one's temper constitute aggression? The problem of definition is important as it affects the classification of aggressive acts, and may lead to misleading findings about the relevance of gender to aggression. Measurements of aggressive responses are also complex – children are often observed for evidence of fighting and other aggressive activity, such as violent fantasy play in the playground; adults, on the other hand, are more commonly involved in a variety of laboratory experiments. Such methods include observing an individual's response to opportunities for verbal aggression, or measuring their willingness to perform potentially violent acts, such as administering (they believe) electric shocks to others.

Since the 1960s, most research has confirmed the view that 'males are consistently found to be more aggressive than females' (Maccoby and Jacklin, 1974). However, since most of this research has been based on children and young adults (due to their ready availability as subjects for psychological research) its limitations must be noticed. Information outside the realms of research, such as crime statistics, does appear to confirm the gender differences in aggressive response, and cross-cultural studies again show that aggression is predominantly a male characteristic (Parkes, 1975).

Biological explanations of aggression

Can male aggression be explained in terms of the biological differences? As we have already seen, these differences are less marked than we might think, but certainly research on animals does show that the male is more aggressive in many species. This aggression is often linked to particular body parts such as horns and antlers, as well as to the male hormone testosterone. As human males also possess this hormone, it may seem a logical conclusion to suggest that this is the reason for the apparent variations in behaviour between males and females. However, yet again, the findings of the established research on animals need to be examined closely, together with the actual link between testosterone and aggression.

Although it is true that many male animals are more aggressive than their female counterparts, many are not, and of those that do support this view, research has often focused on their behaviour during laboratory experiments. Such false conditions may affect the way that animals relate to each other, or the restricted environment itself may cause animals to become aggressive. The animals commonly used for such research are rats and mice, and we might question whether the behaviour of rodents could in any way relate to that of humans. We might also wonder why rats and mice, where there is a distinct gender difference in aggressive acts, are thought to be relevant, whilst hamsters and gerbils, who display similar levels of violence, irrespective of sex, are not.

Many groups of male animals also display violence only at particular times, such as during breeding seasons or to protect their territorial rights. Females too, can become aggressive at breeding times – female mice who are suckling their young are equally aggressive as the males (Archer and Lloyd, 1989).

The role of the sex hormone testosterone also needs discussion. Various studies have linked this hormone with aggression (Persky *et al.*, 1971; Olweus *et al.*, 1980). In the former study, young men were assessed by questionnaires to determine their levels of aggression and hostility, and this was then compared to the rate of testosterone production that each had. The research showed that those males with higher testosterone levels also scored more highly on the test for indicators of aggression. Numerous later studies have repeated this finding, including one, by Ehlers *et al.* (1980) who found that testosterone was also higher in young women with histories of violent behaviour. Does this signify the causal, biological link it seems to represent?

Unfortunately, it is a more complex picture than it appears. High levels of testosterone have also been found in high achievers. Mazur and Lamb (1980) discovered that young men who had won a tennis doubles match for a monetary prize showed a high rate of testosterone production, as did those being awarded their university degrees.

It is difficult therefore to determine the causality of the hormone increase – does it occur as a result of the activity, rather than being the source of the behaviour? Even if the role of testosterone were found to have an influence on subsequent actions, this would not account for the higher levels of aggressive behaviour observable in young pre-pubertal boys, at ages before testosterone has reached any significant amounts.

It is apparent that the evidence for the idea that males are biologically programmed to be more aggressive is less overwhelming than it may first appear. It is also difficult, from the current research, to even show that universally, males are more prone to violent behaviour. However, it is generally agreed that males do commit more violent and aggressive acts than females, and we turn now to sociological explanations of the variations in behaviour between females and males.

Violent men – the roots in childhood?

In order to understand why some men may become violent, it is necessary to consider the socialisation process of children. Primary socialisation, i.e., that which takes place within the family, begins the process of teaching us our gender roles, what is expected of us according to our biological sex. We have already seen how parents may interact quite differently with boys and girls, and there are several other factors which may be influential in children adopting behaviour 'natural' to their sex.

Clothes

Visit any high street children's wear store and you will find row upon row of clothes for girls, whilst there is much less choice for boys, and the commonest boys' clothes are based on football kits, American baseball strips, military style uniforms, or male cartoon characters like Thomas the Tank Engine, Spot, Pingu or Wallace. Certainly the emphasis for boys' clothes is that they are tough, hard-wearing and allow freedom of movement. Girls' clothes tend to be in bright, pretty, jewel-like colours and are often completely impractical for anything other than being admired.

> We go out to buy a pair of summer shoes. I select the ones with decorative stitching that are rather fashionable. The other pairs are quite plain with just a simple leather strap over the instep. Only afterwards does it occur to me that I have chosen the pair that are quite unmistakably girls' shoes. I function like a machine, reacting as expected to the traditional categories: I accept the obvious, as intended. The correct shoes for a girl to wear are the ones that indicate at once that she is a girl. (Grabrucker, 1988)

If we decide to challenge the stereotypical views about what our children wear, we run the risk of singling out our children as different, which they may find uncomfortable. Furthermore, once children are in school, they are likely to be highly influenced by their peers, and want to conform to the prevailing fashions for both boys and girls.

Sigmund Freud (1920/1975) says of woman's need to decorate herself :

> The effect of penis envy has a share, further, in the physical vanity

> *of women, since they are bound to value their charms more highly*
> *as a late compensation for their original sexual inferiority.*
> (Quoted in Gross, 1996)

In other words, females need to look nice to make up for the fact that they have not been born as boys, with all the superiority that confers!

What implications does the choice of clothes have? Firstly, the proliferation of girls' garments gives the message that clothes, appearance and looking nice are important concerns for girl children; whereas boys are not to be interested in looking nice, as long as they can run and jump in their attire. This brings us to the second consequence. How can girls be adventurous, boisterous, climb trees and so on, if they are wearing a frilly dress with instructions not to get dirty? Research by Grabrucker (1988) suggests that girls are more cautious physically, and that this may be as a result of parental expectation as we saw earlier, and also the clothing restrictions we place on them. This female caution appears to be actively encouraged as girls reach school age and participate in sports. Girls play netball, a non-contact sport, similar to basketball (a male game) but which carries much less status, is rarely televised and does not bring sporting heroes to our attention. Many girls do like to play football, cricket and golf, but are rarely able to compete with boys, forming instead all-female leagues. Sports like tennis, athletics, and swimming are segregated, reinforcing the impression that girls are less physically talented or are slower than boys – a curious judgement bearing in mind the wide variations in physique between both boys and girls, especially at puberty.

Toys and books

Both toys and books can be enormously influential in suggesting appropriate roles for boys and girls. Any high street toy shop will be overflowing with prams, dolls that need feeding or changing, pretend make-up sets, fluffy animals, princess costumes that any right-minded little girl would love to own. Similarly, many boys would be thrilled with space crafts, model motorbikes and cars which crash, and virtually any imitation weapon that in real life could cause horrendous injuries – crossbows, sword, daggers, catapults and of course the whole array of imitation guns. It is also the case that girls' toys tend to reflect the domestic life: play kitchens, ironing boards, dolls houses; this can be seen to encourage the nurturing side of their personality, developing skills which it is assumed they will need later on. Boys' toys, however, tend to reflect a world outside of their immediate environment – pirates, space exploration and stunt racing all show possibilities of a wider, more exciting lifestyle. Toys like LegoTechnic are also produced in 'boy' interest subjects, and these together with Meccano, are often thought to develop the spatial and technical skills of boys, leading to the later interest in occupations like engineering, which is still predominantly male. While girls are learning to look nice they are not learning about shapes and form, which may later help with their study of maths. Obviously, boys and girls can be given non-stereotypical toys, and indeed boys' mothers often cite the dolls they have bought their sons as evidence of the unbiased approach they have to childrearing. They also use the subsequent rejection or lack of interest in such dolls as proof that certain forms of behaviour are therefore natural. The parents of girls, similarly, tend to offer little encouragement to them for maintenance or 'fixing' activities, suggesting that it is of no interest to girls to learn how to change a plug or use a drill. Conversely, when small boys help with cooking or even dusting, they are often praised at length, giving them the impression that they have done something really special (Grabrucker, 1988).

Similarly, young people are now encouraged to become computer literate from an early age. However, a browse around any local software retailer will reveal a massive array of games based around violence, death and destruction. The subjects of them are mainly male, often set in futuristic scenarios and always brandishing some form of weapon that can be used to eliminate undesirables. The most popular game to have a female main character is Tomb Raider, but here Lara Croft resembles a male fantasy of what a woman should be like – abnormally slim yet with a heaving breast, incongruously carrying guns. Is it any wonder that young boys are developing computer skills quicker than girls, a fact which again has important consequences for their education? Indeed, technology appears to be unashamedly male and telling us so: consider the Walkman or the Gameboy!

Reading material

Such obvious expectations of gender differences are also apparent in many comics aimed at young children. Most comics which target the under-8 market have a male main character, despite the fact that both boys and girls read them in equal numbers. Postman Pat, Sooty, Spot, Barney, Pingu, Noddy and Peter Rabbit are just a few of them. A comic which has a female main character is usually seen as being exclusively for girls.

Again, girls' comics tend to emphasise either the caring side of their nature, such as Puppy in my Pocket; or reinforce their interest in their appearance, such as Princess, which often offers free gifts of lipstick and nail varnish.

Games

It is not only through the toys we purchase that we may be giving our children an idea of their expected behaviour in relation to their gender. The activities we deem suitable for our children to engage in may also influence their view of what it means to be a girl or a boy. In her diary detailing her daughter's first three years, Marianne Grabrucker (1988) cites many examples of the ways in which we respond differently to children on the basis of their sex.

> We are visiting a friend with a 4-year-old son. The boy is fiddling around with the balcony door, and an argument ensues because he can't close it the way he wants to. Then his mother says in front of both of the children: 'Boys are awful, always up to something. But what can you do about it? Girls are different; they naturally behave more quietly and more sensibly'.

> Of course, girls mess around with doors and do silly things, too – but it's not automatically put down to their sex ... they're just told to stop it. Two hours later, Anneli also has a go at the door. Then our hostess goes across to her, takes her arm, saying: 'Come away from there, Anneli, you might hurt yourself'. (1988:43)

Role models

Parents are the main models of behaviour for many years, so it is not surprising that they have an enormous influence on how we develop a gender identity. The division of labour in the home is still over-whelmingly split on a gendered basis. Despite common perceptions of change, there is much evidence that women, whether in paid work or not, are doing on average three-quarters of the domestic chores (Social Trends ONS, 1996).

More importantly perhaps, is the information discovered by Stephen Edgell in his 1980 research into domestic decision making. Areas such as moving house, car purchase, furniture purchase and food spending were all discussed. Edgell discovered that the more significant the decision (such as moving house or financial matters) the less likely it is that the woman will be involved, whereas decisions about decorating or shopping for food are almost exclusively female domains.

What are the implications of such domestic patterns of behaviour? Simply that girls and boys grow up with an understanding of what is mainly male work and what is female work. Such thinking may lead them to subconsciously form ideas about their later roles within relationships and condition them to accept and indeed expect the very traditional structures that appear to be common in abusive relationships.

'Acceptable' violence?

Another area in which the example set by parents may influence our behaviour as adults, is that difficult issue of discipline. To smack or not to smack? Ninety per cent of parents do smack, with 40 per cent of those feeling guilty about doing so (ICM Poll Chart, *Guardian,* 7 November, 1996).

Many argue that parents have a right to discipline their children in whatever (legal) way they see fit. Smacking is justified as a reasonable force that is used to correct deviant behaviour. This may well be true, and there are thousands and thousands of adults who claim that being smacked in their childhood has not harmed them, indeed it made them aware of their errant behaviour. It therefore serves a useful purpose both for the individual, the family and the wider community. What message is it also giving, though? Most parents would not dream of smacking a teenage son who towered over them. So, we only smack those who are smaller than us. Does might equal right, then? If so, what is the difference between a child being smacked by a parent, and a woman being smacked by her partner? Of course, parents smack their children because they love them, but many violent men also love their partners dearly. Those of us who are parents will be aware of how much our children copy our behaviour. Are we showing them that violence is acceptable if it is done within a family by a close significant other? Are we suggesting that violence is a perfectly acceptable response to both bad behaviour, and also to a person's fragile mood, which is an often mentioned reason for smacking children? If one form of family violence is seen as normal, even desirable behaviour, does this lead to the ambivalent way in which many people think about violence between men and women?

Heroes or villains?

Primary socialisation can be seen to be a powerful process for children, but as we grow older our families exert less influence on us as we are bombarded with ideas and images from a range of other sources, most notably perhaps, the media. We are plied with constant reminders of what the adult female should look like – tall, very, very thin, an object of sexual desire. The waif-like model is used to sell all sorts of commodities – from bathrooms to cars – and such over-exposure of barely clad females may contribute to the way in which women can be perceived as (only) figures of sexual objectification. The controversy surrounding 'Page Three Girls' exemplifies this position. If women's bare breasts are on view every weekday in our most popular national newspaper, does it undermine the status of all women by reducing them to a physical form for the gaze of men? By making women's bodies available to men, are women put in an inferior position in a society that is ambivalent about the domestic abuse of women?

Consider the following celebrities: Paul Gascoigne, Kevin Lloyd, the actor who starred in The Bill until his death, Sean Connery, Frank Sinatra, Stan Colleymore. What do they have in common? All are very successful in their field but all have been accused of behaving violently towards their partners. Is there public outrage about their behaviour? Not really. Have their alleged crimes had an adverse effect on their careers? Not at all. Gazza, whose partner needed hospital treatment for injuries inflicted by him, is still an icon on the football pitch, especially for young fans. He was even named as part of the England National football squad. Ironically, however, the suitability of his behaviour was questioned in relation to the appropriateness of his selection: but it is not the fact that he assaulted his wife that made him unsuitable, but that he had been living it up, 'eating kebabs' and generally acting in ways which may have affected his fitness for the game. Sean Connery has made some very offensive remarks about his 'right' to hit women. What does this suggest about the significance of the crime of domestic violence? It doesn't really matter? It's a private situation between couples, no one else's business? A society which does not loudly condemn perpetrators of abuse and does not show that such activity is completely unacceptable by withdrawing its respect and admiration is really making light of this appalling act. Imagine if a celebrity were found to be a paedophile – would we still be willing to watch them, week after week carving out a lucrative career? Would we be able to put their crimes aside? By our implied acceptance of wife assault, aren't we actually socialising our children to think that it is an insignificant act, a simple explosion of temper, just one of the burdens some women have to bear, particularly if they have behaved inappropriately?

Alcohol and other trigger factors

How we are brought up then, can lay the foundations for how we respond to stressful situations as adults. We have seen that violence may be one such response. Many men, however, will point to alcohol rather than attitude as influencing their behaviour. Indeed, there does seem to be some correlation between drinking excessively and behaving violently, but in fact in relevant studies it appeared to play a lesser part than expected. In the extensive research by Dobash and Dobash (1979) sources of conflict which resulted in violent outcomes were asked about, and alcohol was the sixth most commonly mentioned cause. Similarly, research undertaken by Bourlet (1990) also suggested that while drink could incite violent behaviour, it was a long way down in the list of 'Top Ten' trigger factors. Sexual jealousy is cited as the main reason for violent assault, followed by expectations about domestic work, money and status problems. These causes seem to fit with many of the previously described characteristics of abusers:

– Low self-esteem.

– Belief in the traditional roles of men and women.

– Pathologically jealous.

– Emotionally insecure.

Often, it is a combination of factors which trigger a violent outburst.

Jenny's story (see Figure 2.1) illustrates this point well.

Jenny's story

Jenny was a young woman of 26 who had been married for six years and had three children. Jenny and her husband, Tim, had started off their married life well. They were both working, but Jenny soon gave up as their first child was born. They settled into a traditional division of labour; when Tim came home he was fed, cleaned up after and generally served. Jenny saw this as her role in maintaining their lifestyle – a nice one which Tim worked hard to finance. One day, however, Tim lost his job. They weren't worried at first because Tim was a skilled worker. Another job was bound to come up soon. It did. But it only paid about two-thirds of his previous wage.

Over the next months, they got more and more into debt and began rowing whenever they were together. They could no longer go out much, although Tim still went to the pub regularly with his friends, usually leaving Jenny at home, and returning after she was asleep. One evening, after their usual bad-tempered bickering, they called a neighbour to baby-sit so that they could go to their local pub, where some friends were celebrating a birthday. Once out, Jenny began to enjoy herself. Talking to her friends, she felt more optimistic about her future with Tim. She had a good time, chatting and laughing. She thought Tim was a bit quieter than usual, but she didn't dwell on it. At closing time, Tim hurriedly pushed her through the door and marched her up the road. He was hurting her with his roughness. Jenny, confused, asked him what the matter was. He told her that he was sick of watching her flirting all night, of seeing her laughing and chatting to their friends. He accused her of asking for a wine from their friends, knowing full well that he couldn't have afforded it. She was just trying to show him up. She was a tart. She had trapped Tim. He had never wanted children, he said. They should never have bought a house. What was wrong with a council house like his parents had always lived in? It was all her airs and graces that had got them into trouble. She didn't clean the house properly either. She was just a slut.

Jenny was frightened. She kept on apologising. When they got home, she offered to make a cup of tea, but Tim threw the teapot on the floor and smashed some mugs. They both went upstairs.

As she got into bed, Jenny decided that Tim was stressed about his work and that she must try to be more understanding about how inadequate he must feel. She was about to tell Tim when he struck her with the full force of his fist, on her face. Her nose began to spurt blood but he refused to let her get out of bed. He asked her if she was thinking about Rich, the friend in the pub. She said, of course she wasn't. She was crying. Suddenly he was on top of her forcing her legs apart. Jenny couldn't think straight. He couldn't be doing this to her like this? Eventually, he got off, and told Jenny that neither Rich nor anyone else would want to go with her, she was lucky that he still would. After Tim went to sleep, Jenny got up and cleaned her face. She felt like she was in a dream. She went to sleep at last. In the morning, Tim seemed quite normal. He did apologise for the night before, but suggested that it had been Jenny's fault. He left for work, and Jenny saw to the children. The incident wasn't referred to again, and Jenny began to think it was a complete one-off. I met Jenny in a refuge, about five years after this incident. She had decided to leave then because her children were becoming scared of Daddy, and the new baby made her so tired that she felt she couldn't always be sufficiently on her guard for the wrong word spoken, or the inappropriate look she may give Tim. The violent outbursts had become regular events, and usually coincided with the giro cheque Tim received as his unemployment benefit. On the way back from cashing it at the Post Office he would call in at the pub, returning about teatime.

Figure 2.1 Jenny's story

What was the 'cause' of Tim's behaviour? Yes, he drank excessively on occasion. Yes, he felt inadequate as he couldn't provide for his family. This led him to feeling a failure, and to believe that his wife would leave him. Which of these drove him to violence? A mixture of them all, perhaps. Could Jenny have done anything to prevent all those years of violence?

Whatever we believe about what has led Tim to become an abusive partner, the one thing we know for sure is that it was not Jenny's fault. The responsibility for violence lies clearly with Tim as an individual, and perhaps collectively with all of us as a society.

Can women be aggressive?

The earlier discussion about sex and gender suggested that not only are our gender roles learned, but also that our sex differences (i.e., our physiological characteristics) may be exaggerated. In some other societies, as we have seen, men are men, women can also be 'men', and men can be 'women', if what we mean is behaving in a way which we think of as natural for a particular sex. If we believe that much of our behaviour is learned, it must surely follow that females can learn not to be caring and nurturing (and good at ironing!) but instead learn to be assertive, dominant and even aggressive. Much of the research into crime and deviance amongst young people, appears to suggest that it is only males who commit crime or behave anti-socially. Many of the theories about delinquent sub-cultures focus entirely on the activity of young males. McRobbie and Garber (1977) have questioned whether this was because young women are really not active in sub-cultures, or whether male researchers have made them 'invisible' by ignoring them. Whilst it may be true that teenage girls do not form a large part of male-dominated gangs, this may be due more to the way in which we expect young women to behave rather than to biological differences in their make-up.

Teenage girls are seen as more in need of care and protection; they are more closely 'socially controlled' than boys and allowed out less by their parents, with stricter policing of their leisure patterns than their brothers. Sue Lees (1986) also suggests that young males control the behaviour of teenage girls by the threat of labelling them as sexually promiscuous. It is quite acceptable for boys to 'sow their wild oats', whilst similar behaviour from girls risks them being called 'scrubber', 'slut' or 'slapper'. Against this background of expected behaviour, female sociologists have suggested that the behaviour of girls can be equally as deviant and anti-social as that of boys, but that as a society we are initially more likely to excuse it. If it continues, however, then we find it less acceptable than the equivalent behaviour of males, perhaps because it transgresses our ideas about femininity so overtly. If we consider the incidence of child abuse, for example, it appears that females are responsible for sexually abusing up to 15 per cent of girls in Britain. Jaqui Saradjian (1998), quoted in the *Yorkshire Post* (9 June, 1999), a clinical psychologist, suggests that our society does not like to accept that women can initiate sexual abuse of children, because they are expected to be passive, nurturing and led by men.

Women like Myra Hindley and Rosemary West are often portrayed as more evil than their male counterparts. Is this because their behaviour is so contrary to our perceived view of the 'natural' female personality? Saradjian suggests that many people would feel more compassion to Hindley, if she had stated at her trial that Ian Brady had forced her to join in with his sadistic activities.

This common perception of females as life-giving, mothering and nurturing also often influences us when we think about women, especially pregnant women and mothers, remaining in potentially violent situations with their partners. To some, it seems that they are going against their very nature to risk possible harm to their unborn or live children. Only when we move away from narrow stereotypes will we be able to accept, understand a little, and perhaps offer help to change the difficult decisions made by adult women.

Social construction – myth or reality?

We have looked at the biological and psychological factors which may influence why males and females appear to follow different patterns of behaviour, and we have also considered the various social factors which may contribute to gender differentiated behaviour. When discussing social influences such as role expectation, media images and stereotyping, we have alluded to the 'social construction' of gender, which suggests that the concept of gender and the differences between males and females implicit in the term, are not natural or expected at all, but are in fact derived from or constructed by the society in which these genders are situated. In other words, boys will be boys because we collectively want boys to behave in a way we define as boy-like. Most of us, most of the time, strive to achieve a view of the world that is broadly similar to the way other people around us view the world. So, for example, when the media projects an image of femininity as slim and youthful, many women define themselves against this, and strive to become thinner and keep age at bay. There is no positive image of the older, more experienced woman who ages naturally. Indeed, nearly all women on television (and certainly those in 'serious' positions such as news journalists) are testimonies to hair colouring and personal fitness trainers. Clearly, it is good that we are living longer, healthier lives but do we need to defy ageing or regard signs of it as rather negative? The situation is not quite the same for men, who are often deemed to be eminent, and distinguished and have a lot of creditable experience merely by having grey hair!

CHESTER COLLEGE LIBRARY

The notion of social construction, then, suggests that we make our own reality, but that this reality is usually shared by most other people we respect or are influenced by. Is social construction an essential feature of social life for all of us living in a society? We are obviously all affected by shared ideas and values, but there is evidence that as individuals we can choose whether to accept blanket attitudes affecting our behaviour. For example, within certain limitations, many women can now reject the patriarchal assumptions made about their role within marital relationships. The idea of women's work within a relationship has been dismissed by many, and certainly, those women with educational advantages can fashion a more equal partnership without economic dependence.

Girl power

The current philosophy amongst younger women, too, is that they can lead the life they choose to and can take control of their situation. Decision making and agency have become the responsibility of the individual and there are now considered to be very few societal constraints on how we can choose to live. The Spice Girls have been keen promoters of such 'girl power', but when their image and influence are examined more closely, they appear to uphold the familiar idea of women as being for 'the male gaze', a somewhat contradictory principle to that of 'girl power'. The Spice Girls and similar comparisons have certainly not challenged the idea that looks and sexiness, as defined by males, are important if women want to be successful. More worrying is the impact such role models have had on younger girls – fans are as young as seven or eight. Many pre-pubescent young children are now dressing in 'sexual' ways, copying the behaviour of their elder sisters. Does it matter? It's only fashion after all.

It does matter, though, because young girls are still being socialised into believing that the pursuit of the male is all important, that their likes and needs are secondary, and that, by implication the needs of the male are paramount.

In 1992 Margaret Thatcher said:

There is no such thing as society, only individuals

Has the idea of social construction had its day? Do millions of women feel happy to be married or in long-term relationships? Do they gain immense support, security and happiness from being part of a family? Do they believe they are equal to their partners, and treated as being so? Undoubtedly, the answer is yes to all of these questions. The fact remains however, that roles are negotiated from a position of inequality whether this is recognised or not. K C Backett, writing in 'Images of Parenthood' (1980), highlights the issue of fairness as an important concept that is negotiated by individual family units. The concept appears difficult to maintain, particularly when the issue of parenting arises, where it is frequently understood by both males and females that the lives of mothers will automatically become more restricted than those of fathers. As one woman remarks in Backett's research:

> *The main thing is that he's quite prepared to take charge and give (!) me the freedom if I want to go out; if there's anywhere special that I want to go I know he doesn't mind me going.* (1980:358-360).

Should she be *grateful*? In such relationships, is women's behaviour controlled, not by violence or the threat of it, but by the perceived fairness and equality within the structure? If such principles are genuinely thought to underpin close relationships, are women being 'brainwashed' into continuing to accept a new, mutated form of oppression within marriage? Is 'fairness' then, the new, improved method for male domination?

This chapter has explored the nature of society; we have considered the so-called triggers of domestic violence and the influence of sex and gender on society. We have considered the psychology of gender and asked if male violence is natural. We have examined the various explanations of aggression and looked at alcohol and other trigger factors. In conclusion, we have considered the notion of 'girl power' and dismissed its relevance in the fight for equality and fairness. In the next chapter, we explore some of the issues that define the abuser.

Chapter 3

From all walks of life

He locked me up when I first got pregnant. He didn't think it was his. I told him there was no one else but he locked me in. He's better now. I told his mother but she said I was making it up. I stay away from him when he's cross. He's okay if the TV is on and there is something good on, but he gets fed up of M crying all the time. He is a sickly child. He cries a lot; this gets him going and he lashes out.

As we have already seen, both violent men and abused women come from all sorts of social, educational and ethnic backgrounds. In this chapter, we will be exploring in more detail how a person's background can influence their behaviour as perpetrator, and also discuss how our social positions might affect how we respond to violent assaults from a partner.

Social class

Let us first consider what is meant by the concept of class. Most people would agree that few societies are really equal. Inequalities exist between rich and poor, between women and men, and between black and white. Such divisions are associated with differences in educational opportunities, leisure activities, health prospects, income potential and the power to influence events in society. The stratification into layers or strata is an important starting point for analysing people's behaviour, and in industrial societies like our own, class is just one of the many strata used to differentiate people.

Social class forms an important theoretical concept in sociology, and most commentators accept its existence and significance. As a concept, however, it is extremely difficult to 'operationalise' or use in actual research. A number of different ways for utilising the concept of class have been put forward, most of which are based on a person's occupation. This is because our job is closely linked to the level of income and amount of wealth we have, as well as the skills and qualifications we are likely to have, and the standing we have in society.

Classifications based on occupations include:

- The Social Class Based on Occupation system (formerly known as the Registrar-General's Scale).

- Goldthorpe's model.

- Socio-economic groupings [SEGs].

- Feminist models.

Social classes can be defined as broad groups of people who share a similar economic situation, such as occupation, income and ownership of wealth. In Britain, we are all assigned to the various class groups by virtue of our occupation. Broadly speaking, our job is closely linked to the level of income and amount of wealth we have, as well as the skills and qualifications we are likely to have, and the standing we have in society.

Social Class Based on Occupation system

One of the most widely used methods of classifying people according to their occupation is that of the Registrar-General, who is in charge of the government statistical department, and responsible for carrying out the census and registering births, marriages and deaths. The Registrar-General's Scale uses five main categories of occupation, with a division of Class 3 into manual and non-manual workers, which is also the division between middle and working class (see Figure 3.1).

Social class

Examples of occupation

1 Professional

Accountant, lawyer, doctor, architect

2 Managers

Teacher, nurse, farmer, MP

3a Non manual

Clerical, secretary, estate agent

3b Manual

Driver, bricklayer, hairdresser

4 Semi-skilled manual

Postal worker, bar tender

5 Manual

Labourer, cleaner, refuse collector

Figure 3.1 Social Class Based on Occupation, The Registrar-General's Scale

We can see problems straightaway with classifying people according to their occupations. Why is a solicitor 'higher' than a nurse for example? Who is more valuable to society, an accountant or a refuse collector? There are also differences between occupations in one class: nurses are in the same group as managers and MPs and yet do not normally earn anything like the income of these two. There can also be wide variations within one occupation. 'Farmer', for example, can apply to a wealthy landowner who has extensive acreage of superior quality in a temperate climate; or it can refer to a hill farmer, whose land is mountainous and therefore limited in the amount of food it can produce to feed stock, difficult to gain access to, especially in winter, and above all yielding little in the way of profit.

Another problem is that these class scales are based primarily on the occupation of the 'head' of the household – this is usually assumed to be the man. Whilst this is out of date as so many households have joint breadwinners, it is also sexist and may be a symbol that the woman in a household is actually inferior, despite perhaps earning more, or being in a higher-placed job.

Goldthorpe's model (1980)

This is a more comprehensive system in which there are a larger number of divisions than the previous model. Figure 3.2 outlines Goldthorpe's model

The advantages of Goldthorpe's model are that it:

- Distinguishes between different levels within occupational groups – for example, qualified nurses from auxiliary care staff.

- Clearly distinguishes the self-employed.

- Clearly distinguishes routine clerical workers from supervisors and skilled manual workers.

The disadvantages of using this model are that it:

- Places routine clerical workers above skilled manual workers, despite the fact that the latter may earn more.

– Ignores the very rich and the unemployed.

– Does not reflect the differing female employment patterns.

The service class

1 Higher professionals and managers of large establishments, large proprietors

2 Lower professionals and administrators. Managers of smaller establishments. Supervisors of non-manual workers. High-grade technicians

The intermediate class

3 Routine non-manual workers in administration and commerce

4 Small proprietors, including farmers and small-holders

5 Lower-grade technicians, supervisors of manual workers

The working class

6 Skilled manual workers

7a Semi- and unskilled manual workers

7b Agricultural and other workers in primary industry

Figure 3.2 Goldthorpe's model

Socio-economic groupings

This classification groups together people with similar social and economic status. It takes account of employment status and the size of the establishment as well as the occupation. This measurement more accurately reflects the relationships that can exist in different types of employment, and has been used extensively in research to investigate the links between social factors and life chances.

Many sociologists have defined these traditional systems of classification as 'malestream', in that they are inappropriate for use in categorising women in class groups. Alternative feminist approaches are outlined below.

The individualistic model (Marshall *et al.*, 1988)

Every individual is given a class position based on their present or past occupation. Thus it will allocate 'housewives' to a class according to their previous job. However, can this be an accurate measurement if they have not worked outside the home for several years?

The patriarchal model (Walby, 1990)

This is a complete rejection of the notion that one class model can adequately reflect the differences between males' and females' class positions. The concept of class, according to Walby, implies a common experience, which does not reflect reality.

The cross-class model (Britten and Heath, in Garmarnikow *et al.*, 1983)

A significant number of women in non-manual employment are married to men in manual occupations. The resulting life chances available to such couples are significantly enhanced compared to couples where both partners are located in working-class occupations; and also significantly worse when compared to those couples where both partners work in middle class jobs. This suggests that the nature of the relationship is important, rather than a simple classification based on the (male) head of household.

Alternative occupational categories

In addition to the above models for more accurately assessing the class position of women, some writers have also devised alternative occupational categories, which they claim more clearly reflect this.

Dex (1985) suggests the divisions outlined in Figure 3.3, which can only be applied to women.

Even more radical alternatives have been put forward. Delphy (1984), for example, rejects all schemes which use occupation as a base for measuring class, as she believes that paid work reflects the patriarchal structure in which women are often forced to exist. Such a structure ignores the domestic sphere in which women are exploited for their unpaid labour.

Despite the many problems associated with operationalising the concept of class, it remains a useful tool for measuring the distribution of income and status and their bearing on access to life opportunities in the field of, for example, health, education and housing. A revised classification scheme is currently being devised, which retains some continuity with all of the previous systems of classification, but which addresses many of the problems associated with them (Rose and O'Reilly, 1997). It is hoped that this scheme will be operational from the time of the 2001 census.

I Professional occupations

II Teachers

III Nursing, medical and social occupations

IV Other intermediate and non-manual occupations

V Clerical occupations

VI Shop assistants and related sales staff

VII Skilled jobs

VIII Child care occupations

IX Semi-skilled factory work

X Semi-skilled domestic work

XI Other semi-skilled occupations

XII Unskilled occupations

Figure 3.3 Female occupational categories

The study of class and its links to life chances is invaluable as it enables researchers, Government and society in general to assess whether social changes are taking place; to test the idea that class is in fact no longer relevant. In the area of health, the most comprehensive information about the links between social class and the incidence of illness has been delivered by two influential publications: *The Black Report* (1980) so-named after Sir Douglas Black, but formally known as the *Report of the Working Party on Inequalities in Health*; and *The Health Divide*, published in 1986 but updated in 1992 (Whitehead, 1988). Despite the time between these two pieces of research, their findings are basically the same. *The Health Divide* (1992) confirmed that despite continuing improvement in the health of the nation overall, the gap between classes has continued to widen. Those in lower class/income groups are likely to experience:

- A shorter life expectancy.
- A higher mortality rate in all major illnesses.
- A higher infant mortality rate.
- A higher suicide rate.
- Worse working conditions.
- Lower standard of housing.
- Poorer educational facilities.
- Worse health provision.
- More likelihood of divorce.
- More likely to smoke.
- Fewer natural teeth.

(Townsend and Davidson, 1986)

The 1997 report, re-named *Health Inequalities,* confirmed that the marked socio-economic gradient in mortality and morbidity persisted into the 1990s. In 1998 the Government's independent inquiry into inequalities in health published its report. The inquiry, chaired by Sir Donald Acheson, confirmed that despite the fact that the past twenty years had brought a marked increase in prosperity and substantial reductions in mortality to the people of this country as a whole, the gap between those at the top and those at the bottom of the social scale had widened.

It is difficult therefore to believe that we now live in a classless society. Many people do feel, however, that class is no longer relevant. The main purpose of categorising each of us into a class group is that it enables researchers and governments to gain an insight into the importance of class, and whether significant changes are taking place. For the purposes of this book, stratification into class groups is useful, as it is then possible to discover whether there are particular patterns of behaviour associated with different social backgrounds, and in particular in the way violence between partners is perceived. For many of us, class is a concept which arouses some antagonism, but many people believe that class is no longer relevant.

The expansion in non-manual jobs has led to the enlargement of the middle class. The middle classes value education, have mortgages, spend holidays abroad, and so on – ideas which many of us aspire to, irrespective of our allocated class. One of the factors that has led to higher standards of living for many families is the acceptance, indeed expectation that women will return to paid work after having children, and contribute financially. Since the 1950s, increasing numbers of women have become economically more independent; they enter the public world of the workplace and meet a wide range of people; and they are less bound by the ideas of appropriate roles than their mothers and grandmothers. It might reasonably be expected therefore that the incidence of domestic violence will have receded as women have come to be more assertive and independent. Sadly, the opposite is true – more and more women are reporting violent and abusive incidences, and these figures are themselves thought to be a massive under-representation of the true numbers of such victims. Obviously, the fact that more women are now reporting their violent partners does not necessarily imply that there is more violence in personal relationships, but may be indicative of the fact that it is now more widely acceptable to publicly acknowledge and denounce such behaviour.

So are there any discernible connections between class background and violent behaviour? It would appear from police statistics and records of organisations such as Women's Aid that many more wife-beaters are from lower social classes, but again this may not be a true reflection of the situation. For instance, Women's Aid is an organisation that offers accommodation to women and their children fleeing violence and abuse; those women who seek such alternative living arrangements may be more likely to come from poorer backgrounds without the financial resources (such as a job) to pay for a bedsit or other rented accommodation. Middle-class women may also have middle-class friends or family who have spare rooms where they can stay. Again, figures about the incidence of abuse amongst lower social classes may be misleading, but are there any differences between the type of behaviour, the responses to it, or the possible reasons put forward to account for it?

Domestic violence and the working class

To date, there is no evidence available to suggest that there is any difference in the actual pattern of violence, although it does seem that for families in lower income groups violence is a more frequent occurrence, often almost a means of communication that is 'accepted' by women. Indeed, there is anecdotal evidence that some women who come into refuges have reached breaking point in their relationships but that this is due to a range of factors, of which violence is only one. Amongst this group, violence does seem to be related to external stress such as low income, unemployment, or poor housing conditions. Such pressures may lead to increased alcohol intake, and this in turn may lead to the release of pent-up aggression about the particular circumstances. Stressed, drunk men may lash out at their partners – most of us do vent our feelings on those closest to us. But what leads to the actual violence in such situations?

If we return for a moment to the suggested characteristics of violent partners, we can see that men who feel inadequate, have low self-esteem, or hold traditional views about the roles of women and men, are more likely to beat their partners. No job, no money, and perhaps a wife who is working can all produce feelings of inadequacy in men who have been brought up to believe that they should be the boss, breadwinner and power figure of the household. There is some evidence which shows that men who are unemployed do not necessarily do more chores or housework around the home, even if their partners are working outside the home. This may suggest that such men are rooted in their traditional roles and that any change to these will increase the inadequacy and humiliation they may already feel at being without work or the ability to provide for their family. Do families still exist where the traditional male and female roles and associated division of labour still exist? Indeed they do, and the continual media talk about 'New Man' has served to highlight the disparity between such a figure and the reality for many women. Elizabeth Bott, in her small but influential study of conjugal roles in the 1960s, *Family and Social Networks*, suggested that there were three clearly identifiable types of role:

- Segregated – in which men and women have completely different jobs within the home, for example he does the garden and she does the cooking.

– Complementary – in which partners do related but different chores, for example she washes the dishes, he dries them.

– Joint – in which jobs are allocated according to who can best do them. Both partners can do any jobs as necessary.

Bott's study, which was based on in-depth interviews with twenty families in Greater London, tended to show a relationship between conjugal roles and social class; the most extreme segregation occurred in working-class families. If indeed such a pattern still exists, it may account in some small way for the incidence of domestic violence amongst such a group.

The traditional role of women to service the male head of household, care for any children and fulfil the housekeeping role has certainly been eroded, but for many men who themselves grew up in such an environment, change has been difficult to deal with. In an age in which men were expected to be the main providers for their family, couples were, if not happy, at least accepting of their roles. Over the past two decades, women have been able to venture out from the private sphere of the home into the public world of work. Much attention has been given to their education, with the result that many girls are now leaving school with actual choices about future careers, rather than jobs. A great many women enjoy the opportunity to work outside the home, even though it often entails the 'double shift' of work and housework. Apart from the extra financial independence, they also gain social satisfaction and self-esteem by relating to others; and it is often this new confidence which undermines their partners, for whom the ground is shifting; their wife is no longer the complete doormat she used to be.

Denise, a woman of 34, with two school age children, is typical (see Figure 3.4).

Denise's story

Denise's husband was a train driver, hardworking and a good provider for his family. He was faithful, a good father and his life revolved around his family. Denise had given up paid work after the birth of her children, but had recently found a part-time job as a lunch time supervisor at her children's school. Although low-paid, Denise had wanted to contribute her income to the family, for extras such as a holiday and so on. Her husband was adamant that she use this money for herself, to buy her magazines, clothes and so on. Mostly, Denise spent the money on the children. After some months of supervising school dinners, Denise began to feel a little frustrated. The work was boring, menial and just like the chores she did at home. One day, a friend mentioned she had signed up to do a GCSE at the local college. Denise thought about this for several weeks, wondering if she would be clever enough but also excited at the prospect of doing something a bit daring. Eventually, she enrolled on a GCSE course – one subject over one year. She would have all school holidays off, so she didn't envisage any problems with her domestic arrangements. Her husband, however, reacted differently. In fact he was furious. Why did she need to get a GCSE? Go to college? Mix with students? Slightly confused, Denise started her course, and immediately loved it. She spent ages reading new books, improving her writing skills and thinking and talking about her new discovery of knowledge. She told her husband about all the interesting topics and ideas she was learning about, but he was not fascinated by them in the way she was. In fact, he often ridiculed her, especially in front of their friends. He would say sneeringly that she was trying to become a professor, or he would read out parts of her essays, and laugh about them with his audience. One day, he told Denise that he would buy her the fitted kitchen she had always wanted if she would give up college. But Denise didn't want to.

Some time later, as the course neared its end, Denise began missing lectures, not handing in work. It transpired that her husband, renowned for his temper, had actually begun to hit her. He had become increasingly critical of her performance at home: he said that the house wasn't properly cleaned, the children were being neglected, and he was having to do more domestic work, which wasn't fair after a hard day's work. When she protested he hit her. After the first time, he hit her quite frequently.

Denise didn't complete the course and never returned to college. About two years later, she was seen in a supermarket by a former colleague. She had gained four or five stones in weight, and she had lost her spirit. She had tried to escape the stultifying chains of her expected role, but had failed. Her husband, equally bound by his own expectations, could not readjust to give her some freedom without feeling diminished himself. His frustration had manifested itself in violence towards her, but the long established links and patterns of behaviour between them were more constraining than fear of his strength.

Figure 3.4 Denise's story

Violence in working-class families can be seen, then, as a response to bewildering changes of role and expectation. There is no clear structure or hierarchy any more, and this uncertainty can lead to feelings of powerlessness and loss of control, which can in turn lead to attempts to regain that control, often using violence to do so.

Violence and the middle classes

Is there any difference in the use of violence amongst middle-class families?

There is certainly evidence to show that the 'joint' or 'symmetrical' conjugal role is much more common. Middle-class women are likely to have been educated to a higher level and are therefore likely to be pursuing a career. Although there is still evidence of the double shift amongst dual income families, in that women are far more likely to be responsible for organising child care and housework even if they don't do it themselves, there is an overall acceptance of equality within the home. So perhaps violence is used less as an indication of a power struggle than it can be in working-class families. What psychological purpose can it serve then? According to Jukes (1993), misogyny (the hatred of women) is universal, although as he contends that it is located in the unconscious mind, it is quite conceivable that men 'can hate women without being even remotely, consciously, aware of it' (Jukes, 1993:5). Such hatred informs men's intimate relationships with their partners, and Jukes contends that most men are unaware that anger and tension in such relationships usually arises because women are not behaving in ways which they (men) have defined as appropriate. This perceived failure on the part of women to live up to usually both sexist and chauvinistic expectations, can then lead to abuse and violence in an effort to rectify the situation. However, far from such violence being the result of loss of control, Jukes maintains that it is in fact a demonstration of complete control and manipulation of a situation. Even at the point of violence, men are taking decisions about how to hit, where to hit, and so on, suggesting complete awareness of what they are doing (Jukes, 1993:306). Can this type of analysis have a class link?

The stereotypical macho male, concerned with looking and being 'hard', is more commonly found amongst working-class males. Men from the middle and professional classes appear to be more in control of their base emotions, more placid, particularly in their relationships outside the home. Although statistics show that male against male is the commonest form of violence, this is mostly congregated amongst the lower income groups, where fights particularly among young males, often when alcohol is involved, are not uncommon. Interestingly, police statistics suggest that batterers are actually less socially violent than the male population as a whole, again seeming to infer that battering is not a loss of control, particularly when we consider that such violence is almost always directed towards women in close relationships. So can battering be seen less as a not-uncommon feature of life but rather as an institutionalised response to the incongruity of the behaviour of women as a group? Such an explanation could account more fully for the violent behaviour of many upstanding, respected men who appear to be successful, fulfilled and most importantly, often liked and admired outside their homes. These men are not suffering from the need to project a macho image; they are not experiencing economic or status frustration; they are popular and yet they batter their wives and partners. It is this group of men who appear to be more fully in control, less likely to hit a woman where it will show, and often give the appearance of being a devoted husband to outsiders. Psychological theories are often put forward to account for violent behaviour from such men. Anger is often thought to be rooted in their childhood, or brought about by unresolved family conflict. The modern theory often put forward now is that masculinity is in a crisis, men are threatened by the apparent success of women. Feeling neglected and no longer needed in traditional ways (women do not even need men now to become pregnant!) men have hit back, some of them literally. The violent husband is mad or sad, but not bad. If the man is thought to be emotionally irrational and disturbed, he cannot be fully accountable for his actions. It may in fact be this group of men who are more difficult to help. They nearly always blame the woman for provoking a violent response; and of course it must be recognised that women as well as everyone else can behave in ways which trigger off violent responses in others. However, the decision to actually be violent rests with the perpetrator, and it is this fundamental power struggle that underpins much violence between couples.

Much of the research into abusive relationships has focused on the men and women from lower socio-economic groups. As we have seen, external pressures and other factors such as alcohol are often cited as trigger factors leading to abuse. Where such factors are less in evidence as in middle-class batterers, the approach has often been to label the 'few' deviants as sick individuals who have either learned violent responses from their own disturbed childhood, or have failed techniques for 'anger management'. For all classes, such answers are simplistic and ignore the real issue – that abuse is indeed about control, but rather than being loss of control, it is the actual taking of control over another person, the violated woman. Only when domestic violence is seen as a structural problem resulting from the macro-social inequalities of power, rather than an isolated problem for the individual, of whatever social background, can changes be made to eradicate such institutional bullying.

Violence and ethnicity – 'It's part of their culture'

Women from ethnic-minority cultures are battered and abused just as those from ethnic-majority groups are. Many women, especially those from Asian communities, have been socialised to accept values about their place in society, the irrefutable necessity and strength of the family unit, and above all, the need to accept whatever befalls them without complaining. Thousands of Asian women are brought up adopting these ideas, but that does not make violence and abuse any easier to withstand.

> *The culture into which I was born and where I grew up sees the woman as the honour of the house … In order to uphold this false 'honour' and glory she is taught to endure many kinds of oppression and pain in silence. Religion also teaches her that her husband is her god and fulfilling his every desire is her religious duty. For ten years I tried wholeheartedly to fulfil the duties endorsed by religion. For ten years I lived a life of beatings and degradation and no one noticed.* (Karanjit Ahluwalia, quoted by Kennedy, 1992: 203-4)

Although Asian men are brought up to accept certain marital duties as part of their religious and cultural beliefs, some men ignore or flout such responsibilities. Women in such marriages are often very vulnerable, particularly if they have travelled to Britain to marry, and have no immediate family here. Frequently, such women face deportation if they leave their husbands within the first year of marriage; other women mistakenly believe that the threat of deportation remains in force throughout the whole of the marriage. Asian wives are frequently economically dependent, and are also ill-informed about their welfare and housing rights, with the result that leaving home is rarely considered to be an option. The Asian community, including the religious leaders, and the males of professional classes, frequently side with the husband in an attempt to shore up the institution of marriage. Women who do leave their homes and enter a refuge, for example, know that the whole of their community will be looking for them, and so often the only solution is to move many miles away. Even this, however, does not guarantee safety, with nation-wide networks in place to trace such women. The 'Bounty Hunter' television programme graphically demonstrated how fleeing wives are tracked down through informants throughout the whole country; often these informants are relatives, who believe that community rules must be observed. Efforts are sometimes made to smear the woman's character both as a wife and as a mother – with the result that many women remain in violent marriages in order to keep their children. Asfana's story – an Asian woman with three children – is outlined in Figure 3.5.

Afsana's story

Afsana, a young woman with three children, came into a refuge in fear of her life. She had been beaten with an iron bar, kicked in the head and lost consciousness on at least two occasions. Her sister-in-law rang the Samaritans and the police, expressing concern over her disappearance and demanding that she contact her family if she was all right. The police asked her to do this, to which she agreed, without stating where she was living. An Asian taxi driver was later seen waiting outside the refuge on three occasions. Some days later she received a letter from a solicitor informing her that her husband was seeking custody of the children on the grounds of her unsuitability as a mother. It appeared that he had gathered evidence from a range of community members, including the religious leaders, the doctor and her mother-in-law. The only way to avert this course of action was to return to the marriage. Afsana spoke only a little English, and was not confident that she could exist on her own without family support in another area, so she decided to return home. Some months later she was taken to hospital after being run down by her husband in his car. Despite serious back injuries she returned home without making any complaints and declined offers of support from the refuge workers and police.

Figure 3.5 Afsana's story

Such an outcome does not imply, however, that most Asian women in violent relationships want to remain in such marriages. Asian women, just like any others, want to live in safe environments. They need to know that any action they take will ensure their future safety, and it is this issue of acknowledging the different dangers and pressures on Asian women that is vital in ensuring that women from these ethnic groups have similar options and the right to live free from harm and fear. Indeed, Karanjit Ahluwalia gained two injunctions against her husband, preventing him from entering her house. However, she did not have a telephone and was unable to alert the police when he appeared, and the neighbouring community was unwilling to get involved. This woman was going against the accepted norms of Asian culture. Stereotypical ideas about Asian women really wanting to stay in their marriages must be discarded, if we are serious about confronting domestic violence in whatever community it occurs.

Ethnicity and social class can give no assurances about the safety of women in relationships. Throughout history up till the current day, women from every conceivable background have been subjected to violence in their personal relationships. It is important for us all to remember that we can make no assumptions about the private lives of others; above all, we must always be open to the possibility that one of our friends, a colleague, even a daughter perhaps may be a victim of abuse in their relationships, even though we know them to be confident, assertive women. Even they get battered.

The pregnant adolescent

One of the hazards of writing a chapter such as this is to fall into the trap of perpetuating stereotypes – i.e., a one-sided, exaggerated and usually prejudicial view of a particular group. It would be easy to over-emphasise the experience of domestic violence in a particular class of society or a particular group such as travellers, older or gay women. Stereotypes are dangerous because they are very resistant to change; such views ignore new evidence and create a distorted sense of social solidarity. What we really want to avoid is the belief by midwives that domestic violence is a problem of the poor, the traveller, the woman from an ethnic minority group and not the problem of many ordinary women. The report by Sir William Macpherson on the death of Stephen

Lawrence, a black teenager, shows how the rigid views of one particular group become deeply embedded in the collective consciousness of that group. It seems that many policemen believe, unwittingly or not, that black youths are criminals. This belief, however misguided or distorted, then justifies the treatment of all black youths. Having said that there are specific groups of pregnant women that warrant closer attention and pregnant adolescents appear to be a particularly vulnerable group.

Adolescence is a tumultuous time for most people: the desire to break away from parental control is mixed with a powerful awareness of sexuality and desire to live life to the full. Within the adult, is the child coping with peer-group pressure and struggling to establish individual personal values and identity. It is against this background that the needs of the pregnant adolescent should be considered. Adolescents are both adults and children at the same time. As children they can be abused and as adults they can become pregnant.

It is now recognised that child abuse is a feature of this society and according to O'Hagan and Dillenburger (1995) it is still the problem that has not gone away. However, investigating physical and sexual abuse in children and young adolescents is difficult. Teenagers who are abused may be intimidated by adults, abusive boyfriends, their parents and by their own embarrassment and fear. Parker *et al.* (1994) found that adolescents who report abuse during pregnancy were significantly more likely to have first or second trimester bleeding, gain less weight and report more substance abuse than non-abused adolescents. In another study by Berenson *et al.* (1994) conducted in Texas, 342 pregnant teenagers, aged 17 years of age or younger, were interviewed for a history of assault. Of those who had been physically abused, 40 per cent had been hit during pregnancy. The most common perpetrator of physical assault was a member of their family of origin as compared to a mate (46 per cent versus 33 per cent), although a boyfriend or spouse was the attacker in 80 per cent of cases in which abuse had increased during pregnancy. The face or neck was the most common site of contact, with 14 per cent being hit in the abdomen. These authors concluded that a significant proportion of pregnant teenagers had experienced violence and they felt that this justified the routine screening of this group. It may be that pregnant adolescents, especially those that live at home, are at risk of being hit by both their parents and their partner. Pregnant adolescents may thus be the victims of child abuse by parents as well as victims of assault by their partner. In this study it was the partner that was most often the sole attacker.

In another paper by Covington *et al.* (1997) the researchers report on a study undertaken in North Carolina. The purpose was to determine whether using a systematic assessment protocol could increase the reporting of violence among pregnant adolescents. They found that by using the standardised screening tool there was a threefold increase in the number of adolescents reporting violence during their current pregnancy. The researchers also noted that using examples of specific behaviour rather than vague terms such as violence or abuse resulted in an increase in reporting. They also argued that adolescents do not identify themselves as victims of abuse and often interpreted abusive behaviour as signs of love and commitment to the relationship. It was also found that not specifying the perpetrator of the violence was helpful; this allowed the adolescent to report violence without 'telling on' the perpetrator. Multiple assessments also increase the likelihood of disclosure, especially in pregnancy when the young person may need a series of visits to establish trust and confidence in the person making the assessment. Whilst this quasi-experimental study has limitations, a three fold increase in reporting of violence is important.

In 1998, Curry *et al.* described the incidence of abuse among pregnant teenagers and in particular considered differences by developmental age. In a prospective study, again in America, they defined three stages of adolescent development as early [age 10-13], middle [ages 14-17] and late [ages 18-21 years]. They described the incidence of abuse in each of the stages and found that 37 per cent of adolescents reported abuse, with the middle group 14-17 years, reporting the highest incidence. The 13-14 year olds were most likely to report abuse during pregnancy. Abused adolescents were significantly more likely to experience second trimester bleeding. Although in this study the researchers only screened once during pregnancy, the high rates of reported abuse among pregnant adolescents should ring alarm bells for midwives. Assessment screening is discussed in Chapter 6 but there are lessons for all midwives in these studies. It is very important to avoid assumptions. Some 14-year-old girls will be mature and able to make rational choices and decisions, others will not be. The decision to leave an abusive relationship is a complex one. When the woman is young, single and pregnant the issues are certainly more complex. It would be impertinent to assume that life with an abusive partner is worse than life at home with her parents. Pregnant adolescents should always be allowed the opportunity to talk to the midwife away from their parents or partner. Midwives should remember that adolescence can be a difficult time where criticism or insensitive care will be ineffective. The midwife must always avoid judgmental approaches and take every opportunity to maximise the benefits of antenatal contacts.

Violence and the older woman

The main focus of this book is violence against women of childbearing age, and the image of a typical victim of male violence would probably fit within this age band. As a society we have been slow to recognise that older people, in particular older women, are also the subject of abuse in domestic settings, as well as in the more widely publicised institutional settings. Little is known about what Ogg and Bennett (1992) call 'another iceberg phenomenon'. It is perhaps a reflection of the ageism rampant in our society that the experiences of older women are virtually invisible, apart from the well worn stereotypes about frailty and dependency.

In fact, it is partly the use of such stereotypes that masks the true picture of violence by men against older women. Much attention has been given recently to the plight of 'carers', a largely unpaid and exploited group of workers who provide long hours of dutiful care and attention to (usually) a family member (a spouse or parent) whose physical and mental health is deteriorating. Growing attention is now focused on the stress of providing care in an isolated environment. Whilst such a focus may indeed be helpful, it has tended to overlook that 'the most glaring feature of elder abuse is something that men do to older women' (Whittaker, 1996).

Several types of abuse of older women have been identified, including physical abuse, sexual abuse, psychological abuse, and financial abuse. Within these categories, a wide range of activities has been discovered. Ogg and Bennett (1992) describe enforced isolation, verbal harassment, withdrawal of items essential for living such as heat, food and medicine, in addition to sexual abuse. This last feature creates surprisingly ambivalent responses; sexual intercourse between husband and wife can be seen as just that, a shared intimacy between spouses. However, the question needs to be considered. How realistically can an old woman consent to sexual intercourse if she is suffering from dementia? Can anyone, including her husband, assume she would consent if she was able to?

Can abuse of older women be linked to male violence against women in general?

Clearly, there are a range of different factors to be considered when analysing the many contexts in which older women become the object of violence and abuse. Discourse about carers is obviously a valid addition to the equation. It can be extremely difficult to provide constant, patient and loving care to someone whose needs seem to increase almost daily, and possibly have to readjust to a new unequal relationship at the same time. Women as well as men, are, of course, quite capable of abusing the power invested in them in such circumstances, but the fact remains that only rarely do women engage in either physical or sexual abuse. Such discourse however, draws attention away from the long term violence experienced by many women throughout their relationships and ignores the overriding patriarchal structure within which women exist inside families. In simple terms, getting older does not offer any protection against violence and abuse. Many older women had lived a large part of their adult lives before violence against women had ever been acknowledged. They were, in their isolation, influenced by the many myths surrounding the institution of marriage and their role within it. Many felt that they had 'made their bed, and so must they lie in it'. Violence was for many women only to be expected, after all they had a roof over their heads. If they had wanted to escape from their situation, where would they have gone? Refuges did not exist before the late 1960s, and in any case for women brought up to be completely financially dependent on a man, how would they live?

Florence's story (see Figure 3.6) is one of lifelong abuse.

Florence's story

Florence entered a refuge when she was 76 years of age. She was a frail, rather shaky old woman with quite marked bruising on her face and upper arms. She requested a closer examination of her back. It showed evidence of old beatings, which she confirmed had been carried out with a belt.

Florence had married at 18, and had four children in quick succession. She had never had employment outside the home, but instead spent her time caring for her husband and children. She had celebrated her golden wedding anniversary, before her husband had died six years previously. Beatings and violence had been a regular part of her married life. Her husband had frequently struck her with a garden cane he kept for the purpose; sometimes he had been drinking, sometimes not.

The message was always the same though. Florence was there to take his frustrations out on. Florence understood this. She knew he hated the mill where he worked for over forty years. The work was boring, the wage was low and the noise of the machinery had brought about a loss of hearing. She tried to have everything just right for him when he came home, but sometimes it just was not possible. He would shout at her and eventually hit her, often in front of the children.

The violent behaviour continued after her husband retired, but Florence rationalised that he had become accustomed to this way to let off steam, and she too had become accustomed to it. After her husband's death, Florence felt lonely at first, but she grew contented at the peace she now experienced.

Then her son, in his late forties, asked if he could move back into her house, as his marriage had broken up. Always a creature of duty and loyalty, she agreed. Within weeks her son had taken up where his father had left off. He was angry about his own marital situation and took his frustration out on Florence.

The situation continued for some years, but during these years Florence had to seek hospital treatment for a number of injuries including a broken collar bone. Her son was a much stronger man than her husband had been, and her own physical strength was declining.

An unrelated spell in hospital proved to be the catalyst to allow Florence to rethink her position. Her daughter-in-law visited and revealed that the reason she had left her husband (Florence's son) a few years earlier had been because of his violence. When Florence was well enough to leave hospital, she went to a refuge and contacted a solicitor to start proceedings against her son. He was eventually evicted and served with an injunction preventing him from contacting her at all.

Florence moved back into her own house, at peace at last.

Figure 3.6 Florence's story

In the widening debate about elder abuse, it is very important to retain a feminist perspective so that such violence can be seen as a continuation of the exploitative and violent behaviour experienced by women of all ages. Whilst the obviously stressful nature of caring for older people should be rightfully recognised, not least so that appropriate forms of support can be organised, it is wrong to sanitise violence against older women as a sad but understandable phenomenon. It is not.

Violence in lesbian relationships

In the last ten years, there has been increasing research on violence occurring between lesbian couples (Lobel, 1986; Kelly and Scott, 1989). Generally held opinions of such activity are usually informed by stereotypical views of the nature of lesbians, in that they are often thought to mirror heterosexual relationships – one person (the male/butch figure) dominating the other (the feminine/gentle one). The types of abuse and violence experienced within such relationships are similar to those reported by women in heterosexual relationships, and include physical and sexual assaults, emotional abuse, destruction of property and economic control (Hart, 1986). 'Homophobic control' has also been identified by Hart as an additional abuse in such relationships, by which the violent perpetrator threatens to disclose their partner's sexuality – to 'out' them in fact, to family, work colleagues and so on.

The natural woman?

For many people who are appalled by 'conventional' male to female domestic violence, an alternative type of relationship that seems to escape the usual constructed role restrictions might seem logical. It therefore comes as a shock to realise that similarly oppressive, exploitative interactions occur within lesbian relationships. Such shock depends, of course, on the belief in the influence of biology on personality, as discussed in Chapter 2. Only if we accept that females actually are different from males; are in fact naturally kind, loving and gentle, should we be surprised that abusive patterns of behaviour can occur throughout every type of relationship. We have seen earlier that females can be aggressive, and therefore it is entirely consistent that women can create destructive, harmful ways of interacting with those closest to them, especially if there is an element of inequality within the partnership. The idea that lesbian abuse is somehow 'worse' than heterosexual violence is unhelpful – a 'sliding scale' approach to different oppressive situations does not diminish suffering. If there is a different impact on a victim according to the gender of the perpetrator, it is as much to do with the way society subsequently regards particular acts of violence. Whilst there is usually a lot of sympathy and understanding for women assaulted by men, these emotions are often lacking towards lesbian victims of assault by another women. Little public recognition is given to these survivors, and this feeling of isolation is compounded by the perceived betrayal of a potential ally, particularly if their partner has shared strongly held beliefs about the rights of women.

Linda's story (see Figure 3.7) is about violence within a lesbian relationship.

Linda's story

Linda came into a refuge to escape from her husband with whom she had lived for over twenty years. She had four children, but had only brought the youngest, a daughter aged five, with her. Linda's husband, an ex-army corporal, had frequently lost his temper with her over the years, and his violence had ranged from a slap round the face to vicious kicking, much of it occurring in front of the children. But Linda had remained within the family, mainly because her three older children, all boys, adored their macho Dad and Linda was not confident that she would gain custody of them if she left the household. As her daughter grew older, however, Linda became increasingly aware of the effect the tension and underlying fear of her father was having upon her. Linda left after yet another humiliating beating in front of her teenage boys (who seemed to accept their father's version of why such violence was necessary) and arrived at the refuge in a tearful state. Gradually, she and her daughter came to love the freedom from fear, and Linda decided to seek a divorce. She became more confident and secure by the day, and began giving as well as receiving support from some of the other women in the refuge at that time.

She became especially close to June, a woman in her forties, who was all that Linda felt she lacked. June was quite a strong person who had left her husband of six months after a series of jealous outbursts, culminating with threats of violence and actual physical assault. June had been a shop manager and was comfortable taking control of situations, and to some extent, people. Linda and June's relationship blossomed. Linda admired June's strength – one that she felt she had never had as a woman; June seemed to genuinely care for Linda and her daughter, and enjoyed taking care of them and helping them to organise their new lives. A close relationship developed between them, which quickly became a sexual one. June admitted that she had had several affairs with women previously; Linda was overcome by the love and support June gave her and maintained this by showing June how much she loved her and became paramount to her.

Eventually, Linda and her daughter moved into a new house away from her husband and children, and June moved in as well. All seemed well at first, until some time later, when Linda, in an apparently distressed state, contacted a refuge worker. She explained that the months since Linda had moved into her own house had seen a great change in her attitudes and confidence. She was no longer the cowed wife who did as she was told, who half-believed her husband when he told her that she was lucky he put up with her as no one else would. Linda had emerged from her cocoon to realise that she enjoyed making decisions, could take control of her own life, and had a lot of new opportunities available to her. Linda's growing awareness of her own capabilities was matched however, by June's increasing annoyance and resistance to Linda's ideas.

June appeared to want to remain the dominant, controlling figure that she was used to being, and resented the fact that Linda no longer needed her in the way she once had. Their relationship grew increasingly tense, until one morning, when Linda was intending to enrol for a Further Education course. June had been completely dismissive of Linda's plans, but despite this Linda was determined to develop her educational opportunities, and was in fact excited at the thought of meeting lots of new people and learning new things. Linda's excitement seemed to act as an incitement to June; she raged through the house explaining what a foolish decision it was, and even told Linda that she was not clever enough to study. This comment struck Linda just as though it had been a slap in the face, but she had no time to explore her feelings properly as June's apparently jealous anger escalated, and she flew at Linda violently. In the struggle, June scratched and punched Linda, screaming at her that she was ungrateful, selfish and unwilling to recognise everything she (June) had done for her. June eventually ended her verbal and physical tirade and stormed out of the house. It was at this point that Linda contacted a refuge worker.

Figure 3.7 Linda's story

Some of the characteristics identified by Walker (see Chapter 1) were obviously present in June, just as they may have been in Linda's husband. Joelle Taylor and Tracey Chandler (1995) argue that the issue of violence occurring in lesbian relationships has been used to undermine traditional feminist arguments – if women are as bad as, if not worse than, men there cannot be a valid feminist analysis of male violence. The evidence suggests that it is people who batter and abuse their loved ones, and that such behaviour is more to do with their personalities and backgrounds than the 'natural' proclivities of their gender.

The fact remains that it is overwhelmingly men who batter women. This is possibly because of the whole structure of society – one in which it had been more acceptable and understandable for men to be prone to violence.

Lesley responded to her partner's violence by leaving him (see Figure 3.8).

Lesleys story

Lesley, a woman of 24, had a long-standing relationship with Kenny, 26. They had moved in together nine months previously, after being together for over five years. When they had lived apart, Lesley had thought it really romantic that Kenny always wanted to know about every detail of her day – who she had had lunch with, who was who in her office, and who she danced with on her occasional night out with her girlfriends. After they moved in together though, Kenny's 'romantic' behaviour became, at first annoying, and then rather frightening. Kenny began questioning her about her activities at work; he challenged her about her days out with friends, shopping, unable to accept that she had not met anyone else; and he started listening to her phone calls and asking her what she meant by various comments about colleagues, and so on. His jealously grew worse, and Lesley responded by seeing much less of her friends and eventually gave up her employment altogether when she discovered she was pregnant.

She believed that Kenny would now know how much she loved him and stop feeling so insecure, but in fact, Kenny became even more irrational, telephoning her throughout the day and quizzing her if she had taken longer than he thought fit. On the odd occasion when they went out, he constantly berated her for looking at other men; and if they went out with friends, he spent the evening publicly humiliating her and making fun of her. Lesley told friends he was anxious about becoming a father and also that he was worried about being financially responsible for all of them, although it had been Kenny who had wanted her to leave work.

When Lesley was about 7 months pregnant, a visit to the antenatal clinic, seemingly routine, was the catalyst to the end of their relationship. Kenny started an argument in the car on their return home. He believed Lesley had been 'looking' at the male obstetrician, and that the doctor himself was attracted to Lesley. She accused him of being ridiculous, being ill, irrational. As the car drew up, he almost pushed her out of the door, and into the house. He began slapping her round the face, ignoring her cries.

He left the room suddenly, returning a few moments later in tears himself, begging Lesley to forgive him, and telling her he was scared she would leave him. She said she never would. But the next day, as soon as Kenny had left for work, Lesley packed her bags and left. She had no further contact with Kenny, and she refused to name him on the birth certificate of her baby, in case he traced her. Some years later, Lesley caught sight of him, in a cafe, with a woman and child. The woman looked tired, and unhappy and Kenny was holding her hands as though he wouldn't let them go. She looked scared and trapped.

Figure 3.8 Lesley's story

Violence and travellers

Another ethnic group that we believe it is important to consider is the Gypsies or travellers. We feel this society merits individual attention for two reasons. Firstly, because as travellers, they are often moving around and hence may be outside the normal framework of health care. When such care is sought, it is usually on a temporary basis, such as childbirth, and Gypsy women may not therefore be aware of the help available to them for other situations such as abuse. Secondly, health professionals, like the wider society they are part of, may harbour negative ideas about Gypsies, and this may lead any of us to make assumptions based on prejudice, which are likely to be completely wrong.

The term 'gypsy' is not in fact recognised by Gypsies themselves, who are not an homogenous people but rather a whole myriad of ethnic groups with diverse features. The modern term 'traveller', often thought to be more acceptable, similarly conveys only one aspect of their lives, and again may lead to the formation of mistaken ideas about their culture. However, for the purpose of this book we will examine the most common characteristics of Gypsy life, and hope to lay bare some of the mistaken attitudes they engender, and also show why they are relevant in our discussion of domestic violence in pregnancy.

Gypsies are misunderstood, partly because those who come into contact with them misjudge their customs and in their ignorance project their own insecurities and fears. The Gypsies themselves tend to remain invisible, largely because when they are visible they have experienced stigma and punishment, (such as the ethnic cleansing carried out in Nazi Germany) and such invisibility contributes to the body of stereotypes which abound, often centuries old, but taken as reality by non-Gypsies.

One of the stereotypes that persists is that Gypsies are unclean and unhygenic, and this often feeds into a fear of contamination held by non-Gypsies (Churcher, 1997). In fact, the whole Gypsy culture revolves around the notions of pollution and impurity. These concepts are very much part of the core beliefs that distinguish Gypsies as a separate ethnic group, and despite constant attempts by the wider society of non-Gypsies (Georgios) to become assimilated, they retain spiritual and physical boundaries from the dominant culture.

The relations between the wider society and Gypsies are often focused around the different practices regarding house dwelling and cleanliness. It is often assumed by non-Gypsies that Gypsies would conform to the accepted standards of health and hygiene if washing and toilet facilities were officially provided. Such a view suggests that there is only one set of universally approved standards by which all practices must be measured, with little desire to be ethnically distinct. The complex pollution taboos of Gypsies often centre around the distinction between the outer and inner body – the former is the public self which is presented to society and acts as a protective covering for the latter, which symbolises 'the secret ethnic self, sustained individually and reaffirmed by the solidarity of the Gypsy group' (Okely, 1983:80). The outer body, with its accumulated waste products, is the site of potential pollution; anything taken into the inner body via the mouth must be ritually clean. This applies not only to food but also to cutlery and crockery, which must never be chipped and most importantly must be kept completely separate for the purposes of washing. 'The focus of purity is the washing-up bowl, which should be reserved exclusively for associated activities. The tea towel must be washed in this bowl and never with the laundry. The tea towel hanging out to dry on its own becomes the symbol of ethnic purity' (Okely, 1983:81).

The focus on the complete separation of various activities contributes to the suspicion held by both Gypsies and non-Gypsies towards each other. Gypsies regard the non-Gypsy tradition of indoor toilets as completely polluting, by situating defecation and urination areas close to food and domestic quarters; whereas for Gypsies such polluting dirt may be visible, for example done in a field, but must be some way away from the home.

Such major differences in the way of life and the symbolism attached to various activities are obviously a cause for potential conflict when

Gypsies are obliged to enter the non-Gypsy world, such as when they need hospital treatment. Indeed, hospitals are often regarded as the most dangerous of places, as they combine suspect cooking and cleaning practices and are seen as places of disease. Gypsies often resort to hospitals only at certain times, one of which is childbirth, which is seen as a polluting act. Against this background of fear and suspicion, it is clear that the role of the midwife is a very difficult one. They must not only overcome their own feelings of distance and difference, but they must also try to recognise whether any views they have formed are rooted in reality or are based on a set of faulty assumptions. The Gypsy woman may appear frightened, nervous, even distressed, but this may be due to her fears of being in an alien environment, rather than be related to her personal home circumstances. An awareness of the probable reasons for a Gypsy woman's apparent anxiety however, must not obliterate the need to think about the possible reasons for such emotions. As we have seen earlier, there are few known societies in which domestic violence does not occur; therefore we can safely assume that Gypsy culture is also likely to be party to it. If we examine the structural relationship between women and men in Gypsy culture, we can see that they occupy different positions within their society, and are subject to very different social sanctions. Such differences may explain Gypsy women's vulnerability to violence in the same way as it may partly account for the threat to women in the wider society.

The dominant, non-Gypsy society often portrays Gypsy women as alluring, tempting sexual creatures. Indeed, the main character in the opera *Carmen* (Bizet) is always played as a black haired, voluptuous figure with full hips and a provocative walk. In reality, the sexual activity of Gypsy women is carefully controlled; they must remain a virgin until marriage, and were traditionally inspected by older married women to confirm this. Sexual fidelity is essential after marriage, and Gypsy women are even wary of being seen in conversation alone with a man other than their husband. They are subordinate to their husband's wishes and must observe strict rules regarding their dress and manners. Despite having the main responsibility for children and the domestic chores, Gypsy women are also expected to work for financial gain outside the home, in contrast perhaps to the relationship of some women to the economy in the wider society. The work that Gypsy women are engaged in usually involves 'calling' at the houses in the area selling small items such as tea towels.

The reason that Gypsy women are thought to be better at this activity shows a keen awareness and indeed a manipulation of the prejudices often held by non-Gypsies. As women in the dominant culture are not normally expected to be the main breadwinner, so Gypsy women are also regarded as economically dependent on their husbands, and indeed often pose as 'an abandoned, near-destitute wife and mother'. By eliciting the pity of the Giorgio, she can extract a greater economic return (Okely, 1983:204). Certainly in the past, the Gypsy woman was almost entirely responsible for the purchase of food and domestic requirements.

Maybe it's not like it used to be, but in the old days a Traveller's wife had to work. Otherwise they'd beat them.

Although Gypsy women have often been expected to provide the subsistence requirements, they are rarely able to purchase or own capital items such as trailers, cars or horses. As we have seen, economic dependency can often be a factor in a violent relationship, a symbol of power and control.

As we have said earlier, the period during and after childbirth is regarded as a time of great potential pollution. The almost universal preference for Gypsy babies to be born in hospital has tended to be misinterpreted as an acceptance of the dominant culture's values and advice. In fact, removing birth to an outside environment is seen as a way of limiting the potential contamination of dealing with polluted items, by allowing others to handle 'unclean' items such as towels and bedding. Time spent at the hospital is kept to an absolute minimum; antenatal care before the actual birth is not widely regarded as necessary, unless it is seen as a way of ensuring access to a hospital bed. Similarly, Gypsy women often discharge themselves immediately after the birth. Such an apparently disdainful regard for the services of the health authority and, in particular, midwives can lead to negative feelings being experienced by the health professionals concerned. It should not be seen, however, as a personal rejection of the care offered, but rather as a clash of cultures in which expectations and understanding of behaviour vary widely. Obviously, an appreciation of Gypsy culture and the symbolism surrounding childbirth are vital if the needs of the mother and her baby are to be met; if there are additional problems, such as domestic violence or abuse, these can then be more easily identified.

If a Gypsy woman appears to be the victim of domestic violence, do non-Gypsies have the right to intervene in a social structure that they may not fully understand? Of course not. Neither do they generally have any power to do so. What midwives and others can do, however, is to ensure that possible victims can have access to sources of information and support, and also the knowledge that alternatives are available.

So why should anyone stay?

In this chapter, we have seen how violence and abuse against women occurs throughout the social spectrum. There appears to be little correlation between class background, age or ethnicity and even sexual identity, and the risk of experiencing violence. Even being male does not completely erase the risk. What all these people (overwhelmingly women, of course) have in common is that either emotionally or financially, they are in relationships of unequal power, in which they are the more dependent. Such dependency may result from the wider economic structure, or from a psychological dependence that is learned by most females from an early age. Whatever the cause, the consequences are the same. Women, often mothers, believe that they need a man to take care of them and their children. Any relationship is better than none, especially if the man is the father of their children. If women fulfil their side of the bargain properly (as defined by males) then they will be cared for. If they are then abused, most women search themselves for the fault they believe has led to violent behaviour. Many of the stories in this book make horrific reading and appear unbelievable. Sadly, they are all true. Despite the appalling suffering, many of those women remained in those relationships for many years. Why? Precisely because they were financially or more importantly, psychologically dependent, or believed they were. If women are living with the fathers of their children, there may be a lot of guilt about taking them away from a father who may be loving and generous to them. If children are older, there may even be a worry about whether they will want to stay with their father, leaving a woman alone and lonely. There may also be worries about coping as a lone parent, dealing with the practicalities as well as the emotional problems that may ensue. Years of abuse, mental cruelty and violence do not do much for one's self-esteem. Indeed, being beaten, belittled or blamed constantly can only lead to complete loss of self-worth and feelings or complete inadequacy. Many people will have had experience of being criticised, perhaps at school, or in a work situation, and know that it can lead to a loss of confidence. How much worse then, if the criticism comes from someone you love. You have been so bad, that the person you care about most, is angry with you – it must be your fault. When this attitude develops, it becomes hard to think dispassionately about the situation. Seeking help means that personal faults will have to be revealed to others, who may in their turn (the thinking goes) be equally disappointed.

The question we need to ask is not: 'Why don't they just leave?' It is: 'How can we help women in violent relationships?' We can give them information, encouragement, sympathy, but most of all we can give them understanding that the choices they have to make are difficult ones. We who are lucky enough, (and yes, it is luck at stake), to live in violent-free relationships, above all must not judge the actions of those who do not have such peace. These issues are explored in more detail in Chapter 6.

In this chapter, we have considered how a person's background can influence their behaviour as perpetrator and individuals' responses to violence. We have explored the concept of social class and considered the difficulties that surround the classification of individuals. We have debated the issues around domestic violence and working classes and challenged some of the stereotypes that are perpetuated in health and social care. We have discussed domestic violence, the middle classes and the issue of ethnicity. We have discussed the adolescent, the older woman, women in lesbian relationships and travellers. We have concluded the chapter by beginning the discussion around why anyone should stay in an abusive relationship. We will consider this issue further in later chapters.

Chapter 4

The underlying causes of violence

*If it is not safe to let oneself be dominated, then
it is not possible to be fully feminine*

(Anthony Storr in *Women in Human Aggression*, 1970)

*Another black eye and a few broken ribs are, of
course, just the thing to make a woman feel
deliciously feminine.*

(Elizabeth Wilson on Anthony Storr in *What Is To Be Done About Violence

Towards Women?*, 1983)

In this chapter, we peel back more layers of the onion. We explore the underlying causes of violence and explore some of the established feminist theories. We explore the concept of a continuum of male violence and ask if feminist theories can help. We explore the powers of the professional and the impact of professionalism on child-bearing women.

In the previous chapter we have looked at the some of the most observable causes of domestic violence between women and men. Factors such as jealousy of another person (adult or baby), feelings of inadequacy, or external factors such as unemployment and financial worries can all lead to sensitive situations, which may erupt into violent confrontations. Perhaps many of us can, if not condone such behaviour, at least understand it somewhat, especially if we connect to the experiences of parents who may lash out at children, often regretting it afterwards. However, whilst domestic violence is relatively common (a survey carried out for the Granada TV programme *World In Action* (1989) suggested that one-third of all married women had been the victims of violence from their husbands) such violence is almost always perpetrated by men on women. As we have seen, the size and shape of males and females is variable, therefore the pattern of violence cannot be claimed to be exclusively concerned with physical might. Why then, do thousands and thousands of men react to stresses by beating their partners? In this chapter we will be considering the underlying power structure in society, by which men both as individuals and as a social group, assume superior positions over individual women and women in general. We shall also review the role of feminism in raising awareness amongst women and men about gender divisions. We will be using the major feminist theories to try to make sense of not just the violence inflicted by one individual on another, but to extend our understanding of the social and economic context within which violence takes place.

The social movement known as feminism is by no means a modern one. Women throughout history, in all societies, have declared their resistance to being treated as a subordinate class. Mary Wollstonecraft wrote a treatise entitled *A Vindication of the Rights of Women* in 1792, in which she maintained that inequalities between men and women were not the result of biological differences, but were due to environmental differences, especially the fact that women were excluded from education. Wollstonecraft argued that both women and society were damaged by the limits that women were conditioned to accept. Nineteenth century feminism was concerned with women having the same legal rights as men. Women did not gain the right to divorce on the same grounds as men until 1934; prior to that time, women who were separated from their husbands had to rely on relatives to keep them . They were denied a right of access to their children in the case of marital breakdown; a right to control their own property, including jewellery and clothing; and a right to their own earnings.

Nineteenth century feminists were also active in the field of sexual exploitation. They believed that increasing sexual liberation for men resulted in increased oppression for women. The increase of the female age of consent from 13 to 15 was an example of the perceived need to acknowledge and establish the separate sexual needs of women from those of men. Indeed, prior to this time, women were not thought to have any sexual interests whatsoever, but merely to be passive recipients of their husband's desires.

Twentieth century feminists have both extended the focus of women's rights in the public sphere, and also developed an analysis of women's role in the private sphere of the family. Since the 1960s, feminism has often received a bad press, and has occasionally alienated both men and many of the women whose cause it sought to champion. The reasons for this are complex. Whilst it may be quite understandable that those whose privileges may be affected would not support the ideas propounded by feminists, it must be less clear why those who stand to gain from feminism's success also often reject it. Many feminists themselves believe that this is because the level of brainwashing or conditioning is so pervasive that it is difficult to recognise, let alone consider changing, the nature of society. Whilst individual women and men may struggle with the realities of inequality, poverty and discrimination, it is difficult to stand back from day-to-day tribulations to recognise that society itself may be structured in such a way as to create structural injustices. Indeed, feminists themselves, whilst being able to recognise underlying processes of inequality, do not share an homogenous view of the causes of such inequality. In the last thirty, or so, years, several different theories of feminism have been developed, the most popular among these arguably being liberal, Marxist, black and radical feminism. We need to consider all of these briefly, in order to measure to what extent they are able to account for the continuing oppression of women by men, especially in the form of domestic violence.

Liberal feminism

Liberal feminism has its roots in the liberal tradition of the Enlightenment, which stressed the principles of justice, rationality, citizenship, human rights, equality and democracy. Liberal feminists believe that as rational beings, women should be entitled to the same legal, political, social and economic rights and opportunities as men. They recognise that women are occasionally discriminated against because of their sex, and that much of this discrimination is informal, based on custom, the product of sexist assumptions, which are the product of gender role conditioning. For liberal feminists, political action and reform are the key to addressing inequality, with the emphasis on educational strategies and legislative changes, and with the aim of both providing women with opportunities and challenging stereotypes and prejudices. According to this explanation, then, gender divisions exist because we do not have equal opportunities. They exist because of individual prejudice and discrimination, and because through sheer unenlightenment, the opportunities open to men have not yet been extended to women. Legislative measures such as the Sex Discrimination Act 1976, and the Equal Pay Act, and educational changes such as the National Curriculum have given women more equality, and have challenged entrenched attitudes to some extent. However, if we look more closely at the current position of women, we can identify major weaknesses in the liberal feminist theory. Firstly, the idea that discrimination is solely to do with individual attitudes, which can be changed, ignores the question of why such attitudes exist in the first place, and why they are maintained. The legislative changes that have taken place certainly have had some impact on the lives of women. In the public sphere, opportunities have opened up for women: they are spending an increasing proportion of their lives in employment, although very few have continuous full-time careers because of their domestic responsibilities (Martin and Roberts, 1984).

In Britain, over half of employed mothers have part-time jobs. However, studies such as those carried out by Susan Yeandle (1984) and Judith Chaney (1981) show that women in Britain search for jobs that they think appropriate for their domestic situation – this is often part-time, low paid work such as school-meals supervisor, shelf-stacker and checkout-operator.

Employers also have a clear idea about what is appropriate work

for women, and they seek to 'activate' a supply of female labour.
(Abbott and Wallace, 1997:209)

It still remains true, sadly, that many employers are more reluctant to employ mothers than any other group, because of fears that they will have to take time off to look after their children when sick. Also, the feeling still persists in some quarters, that mothers are likely to be less committed to their jobs because of the role conflict they may experience; their families will always come first, so they will therefore be less flexible to the needs of the workplace. In a society in which the care of children is still seen as predominantly woman's work, it is not surprising that women do seek jobs that allow them to fulfil these domestic functions as easily as possible. In this way, despite legislation, opportunities for women are not equal; they are restricted in the hours they can work, and are therefore also penalised in the wages they can earn. Companies know that they can get plenty of female workers to work for £3.00 per hour, so why pay more? Indeed, the new legislation concerning minimum pay will mainly benefit women, as it is mainly they who are working for less than this amount. We can see that if women are actually congregated in jobs that traditionally offer low pay, then this will negate the supposed benefits of the Equal Pay Act, which states that women should receive equal pay for work of an equal nature. This is because there will not be many males working in equivalent jobs in many of the areas that are thought to be 'women's work'.

Similarly, despite educational reform, although girls are either matching or outstripping boys' performances in most GCSEs, they are still less likely to go to university, and if they do, girls are more likely to choose subjects regarded as lower status, such as language and literature courses. Reasons for gender-related subject choice cannot simply be addressed by equal opportunities policies; whilst these may make it possible for girls and boys to choose whatever subjects they wish to study, the force of socialisation and peer-group pressure still exert tremendous influence. Also, despite the statistical data showing changes in the overall achievement of girls and women, gendered messages are often transmitted through the curriculum content, or through the choice of text books, or through interaction with teachers, many of whom are completely unaware that they may be treating boys and girls differently.

We can see from the examples of work and education that the liberal theory of feminism can be used to develop strategies and political policies that will at least make people aware of discriminatory practices. The past one-hundred years have seen women gaining increasing equality. How, though can the liberal feminist theory be used as an explanation of domestic violence? True, it can raise the legal profile of battered women, although to date the general public tends to be more outraged by the murder of an innocent man by a schizophrenic who has been the victim of inadequate community care, than the reported beating or even killing of a woman by her partner.

It fails though to suggest reasons why men should hit women in the first place. Clearly, they do not 'need' to hit them in order to be superior: they already are – women have needed to resort to the law to ensure at least some degree of equality. What is missing from this theory is some attempt to understand why men systematically hold power over women, and why this power is:

> *embedded in, and reinforced by, all the institutions and organisations of society, and the way it operates regardless of the wishes or actions of any one group or individual.* (Wilson, 1983)

Marxist feminism

In an effort to address the wider context of male power, Marxist feminism has developed a theory to account for the subordination and exploitation of women in capitalist societies. Central to capitalist ideas is the need to make profits and produce wealth. The organisation of production and the division of labour are fundamental to wealth creation, and it is this relationship to the workforce that determines the level of exploitation experienced. Many Marxist feminists argue that women are kept in a weaker position because of their relationship to 'reproduction'. This term has two distinct meanings from this perspective. Firstly, there is the obvious one that women are the childbearers and as industrialisation came increasingly to separate home from work, a distinction between the private domestic sphere and the public world of work became apparent. Women are useful to a capitalist economy because having other domestic responsibilities often means, as we have already seen, that they are willing to take on low-paid jobs that fit in with family life. They are regarded as a flexible labour force, or as Marxist feminists claim 'a reserve army of labour', taken on when consumer demand is high, and laid off when there is a slump. A clear example of this occurred during the Second World War, when women were desperately needed to maintain the manufacturing industries, and all thought of whether it was good or bad for children to have working mothers was dismissed. After the war, when returning soldiers needed their jobs back, many women were forced back to the home because the government-run crèches were shut down. Thus women are an easily disposable workforce who can be reabsorbed into the home, without even, until recently, featuring in the unemployment figures. So women can reproduce, that is bear and rear children who will themselves grow up to be the future work force; but they also reproduce the status quo, by servicing the current work force (that is, their husbands) through all the domestic activities which make up housework, as well as through the emotional and sexual duties that wives perform. This nurturing role is useful to capitalism because it ensures by and large a happy, satisfied workforce who are motivated to work hard to support their families.

This vital work is also unpaid! Any change to the powerlessness of women can only (from this view) be accomplished through a complete change in the economic structure of capitalist societies.

Clearly, the Marxist feminist arguments about the necessary division of labour appear to be valid. Women are valued according to their worth to the economy; therefore educated women can expect to have good jobs, but can also often expect to have to do what is called the 'double shift' – namely bear the main responsibility for the domestic organisation of their homes and children, even when they are in full-time employment. The fact that thousands more women are now in the workforce can also be understood in Marxist terms; the economy has expanded and needs a much larger workforce than can be met by current workers and school leavers. There are, however glaring weaknesses in the argument. Firstly, the theory suggests that capitalism is to blame for the weaker position of women. If this were the case, we would not expect to find gender divisions in societies that are older than capitalism, or which have never been capitalist societies. Sadly, this is not the case. In Ancient Greece, the birthplace of democracy, 'everyone' had a vote except slaves, and of course women. In communist Russia, women usually did have paid employment, but were also held responsible for all the domestic chores at home. Most importantly, even if we accept capitalism as a cause of gender division in the workplace, what relevance has this to understanding why men beat their wives, why pornography exists, or the extent to which women have been marginalised in other spheres, such as the Church, or the Arts, neither of which have much to do with the means of production?

Black feminism

In recent years, black feminists have begun criticising what they regard as ethnocentric theories that ignore the particular experiences of black women (Anthias and Yuval Davis, 1993); and many suggest that looking at the world from a black woman's perspective brings new insights into social relations (Hill Collins, 1986). The relationship between white women and white men is not the same as that between black women and black men, but as Joseph (1981:101) suggests:

> *capitalism and patriarchy do not offer to share with black males the seat of power in their regal solidarity ... there is more solidarity between white males and white females than there is between white males and black males.*

Black women share with white women a history of oppression, and they also share with black men a history of racialisation. Working-class black women and men are subject to economic oppression, racism and discrimination and many within that culture may believe that the racially oppressive context in which black people live is a contributory factor to the violence within families, against women. Clearly, however, such oppression is not the only causal factor in wife beating, as many oppressed men do not become abusive, and furthermore, many

> *powerful and privileged men also abuse and torture the women they have relationships with, often in even more premeditated and sadistic ways.* (Mama, 1989:302)

The need to recognise that the experience of black women is different from that of white women is therefore, central to the arguments of black feminists. The Southall Black Sisters have suggested that black women have to struggle against cultures and traditions that keep them weakened and without the power to determine their own lives. They insist that white feminists should accept the differences between them, and struggle alongside them:

> *Why is it if a white woman is killed as a result of domestic violence it is an issue for all feminists; if a black woman is killed it is an issue for black women only. It is as feminists, not as white women, that we ask you to participate in this action. Until you see the struggles of black women against oppression as your struggle there can be no basis of solidarity between black and white women.* (Quoted by Pearson, 1992:268)

An example of this distinction between apparently similar experiences can be seen in the case of Karanjit Arowahlia, an Asian woman who was convicted of the murder of her husband, a man who had violently abused her for years. Although her case received some publicity, it was nothing compared to that given to Sara Thornton, also convicted of murdering her violent partner, but a white, articulate woman whose case was used to call for changes in the law due to reasons of provocation. She was a universally acceptable figure, whilst it was feared that Karanjit Arowahlia, with her traditional Muslim dress, and her limited English, would marginalise the campaign into a black issue.

This is a clear illustration that white experience is perceived as the norm, black experience is the 'other'. This concept of the 'other', which does not form part of mainstream knowledge, is part of what Barker (1981) calls the new racism. No longer can groups be differentiated and discriminated against on the basis of their race as a marker of biological inferiority; this has been discredited, and there is no evidence that biological differences affect social behaviour. The new racism, according to Barker, talks about cultural differences, and perceives these as a problem, especially where people with different cultures live in the same location. There is complete belief in the idea that there is a dominant culture to which most people (all white) belong. This idea of homogeneity is a curious one when we reflect on British history, and realise that our island has experienced mass immigration, both peaceful and as a result of invasion, on several occasions, bringing new cultural groups to our lands on each occasion. The dominant (British) culture has historically included the Romans, the Vikings, the Celts, the Angles and Saxons, and the Normans, to mention but a few of our fair-skinned ancestors. Is it possible to extract a solely British character? From a contemporary perspective, how much of our culture has been expanded by the immigration during the past forty years of people from the continents of Asia and Africa? The explosion of Chinese, Indian and Caribbean restaurants has changed 'British' eating patterns permanently, and the contribution to sports, athletics and football in particular, by those from different ethnic backgrounds has helped to develop a collective pride in our sporting achievements. To suggest that the likes of Andy Cole, Frank Bruno, Denise Lewis or Linford Christie are somehow not part of British culture, but form an 'other' cultural group with different loyalties is clearly at odds with the immense pride they all demonstrate when representing England or Great Britain in their field.

Similar assumptions and stereotypes towards black women must also be recognised and countered. The issues of violence against those from African and Caribbean origins tend to focus mainly around perceived police brutality rather than violence against women by their partners. In fact, black women's oppression has often been understood in terms of the fact that:

> black men beat black women because they themselves are brutalised by state repression. (Mama, 1989:84)

Mama also suggests that:

> high levels of violence and cruelty to women, by the men they are, or have been, in relationships with, are being tolerated by the communities themselves, as well as by statutory organisations.

This attitude of acceptance of family violence within the black community is obviously likely to influence other agencies such as the police. Research suggests that 47 per cent of those women interviewed by Mama (1989) had never contacted the police, even though most of them had had to leave their homes because of the violence and had become homeless as a consequence. The negativity sometimes shown by the police towards black people itself generates a negativity from them towards the police – a complete lack of confidence that police involvement would aid their situation.

Radical feminism

The starting point for this theory was in the early 1970s, with the 'second wave' of feminism. Although radical feminists agree with the Marxist view that gender divisions are concerned with power and oppression, they do not share the view that such divisions are related to class and capitalism. The key concept in radical feminism is patriarchy, rather than capitalism. Using this concept, unequal gender divisions can be accounted for by the way in which they serve, not the interests of a capitalist society, but the interests of men. Kate Millett, in her ground-breaking book *Sexual Politics* (1970), describes patriarchy as:

> *What goes largely unexamined, often even unacknowledged in our social order, is the birthright priority whereby males rule females. Through this system, a most ingenious form of 'interior colonisation' has been achieved. It is one which tends moreover to be sturdier than any form of segregation, and more rigorous than class stratification, more uniform, certainly more enduring. Sexual dominion obtains as perhaps the most pervasive ideology of our culture and provides its most fundamental concept of power.*

This is so because our society, like all other historical civilisations, is a patriarchy. The fact is evident at once if one recalls that the military, industry, technology, universities, science, political office and finance – in short, every avenue of power within the society, including the coercive force of the police – is entirely in male hands (Millett, 1970: 24-5).

Patriarchal society

According to Millett, patriarchy is universal. It characterises every known society. Patriarchy exists not just in people's experiences, but also in their heads – it is the norm. It is a systematic set of social relationships through which men dominate and maintain power over women. The relatively few individual women who have achieved decision-making posts in whatever field make no difference to the overall structure of male-dominated society.

Millett and other radical feminists do attempt to explain why and how men have acquired this power, unlike the previous feminist theories. They believe that the reproductive system of women has made them dependent on men. Until quite recently, women in all societies have spent a lot of their adult life bearing children, and many believe this has enabled men to take control in all major public spheres, and often in the private spheres as well. Even in our society, where childbirth is no longer the dominating activity of a woman's life in terms of the years spent in pregnancy, the technology surrounding birth control is in men's hands; and men occupy the most powerful positions in all medical specialties, including obstetrics.

Radical feminism then, can begin to account for male violence towards women by suggesting that violence, or the threat of it, is one way in which men retain their control over women. The fact that men dominate both private (family) and public (work, and so on) spheres shows how powerful the ideology of patriarchy is. Most of the time we do not even question clearly unfair situations such as the loss of female freedom when a rapist is at large: women are advised not to venture out at night and definitely not alone. It is a man who has committed the crimes against women, and yet it is the civil liberties of women that are withdrawn. Surely, it would make more sense to curtail the freedom of men, one of whom has committed rape? A similar situation occurs when a man has been involved in a violent outburst against his partner – very often, the police will bring a woman and her children to a refuge in the middle of the night, whilst the violent offender is allowed to remain in the familiar surroundings of his own home. This is part of the 'interior colonisation' that Millett speaks of, situations so commonplace that we cannot for the most part recognise that they defy meaning or rationality.

Radical feminism accounts for domestic violence as a tool that reminds women of their place – subordinate. The fact that not all women are in, or have been in, an abusive relationship is immaterial. All women know that this is possible, and it is this eternal threat which keeps women scared and broadly compliant. As Stanko (1985) says:

> The brutal rape, the sexually harassing comments, the slap on the face, the grab on the street – all forms of men's threatening, intimidating and violent behaviour – are reminders to women of their vulnerability to men. Try as they might, women are unable to predict when a threatening or intimidating form of male behaviour will escalate to violence. As a result, women are continually on guard to the possibility of men's violence.

The fact that many abused women actually do excuse their violent partners, is testament to the fact that domestic violence is seen as 'acceptable' or understandable by women themselves.

Radical feminism then, purports that men have taken control of all the major areas of public life and also exercise a large degree of power in the private institution of the family, as suggested by Edgell in his study on decision-making in the home (1980). Men are in charge in our society:

> *not only do they hold the most influential positions and own and control most of the resources, but their positions and resources enable them to be the 'experts' who make pronouncements on what makes sense in society, on what is to be valued.* (Spender, 1982:5)

But why does such a differential in the power base lead to violence? It may be understandable as a means of protecting the status quo, enabling men to hang on to their power and privilege. Although only a minority of men are violent in their personal relationships, the rest are linked with this sort of expression of control by association: the risk for women is always there, always a possibility. As we have seen, the lives of women are often constructed through their relationships with men; women are unwise to walk in certain places at certain times; must dress 'appropriately', so they cannot be accused of 'asking for it' if they are raped, and must often put up with harassment at work or risk being sacked. Violence is the ultimate deterrent, and fear of violence is equally powerful.

Radical feminism attempts to explain why patriarchy has existed so successfully for so long. As humans we are born into a patriarchal society; we must be socialised into the ways and thinking of this society in order to become proper members of our community. However, the ways and thinking, the words, language and concepts which we are all socialised into accepting, are ones

> *developed by males and in which male power is promoted and justified. Having been socialised into a patriarchal society, our vision is circumscribed, our possibilities for envisaging and explaining an alternative are limited.* (Spender, 1982:10)

It is difficult to imagine how a patriarchal society could identify, let alone seriously consider, that the power yielded by men is a central problem for women. Patriarchy is thus a self-generating concept.

We can see how such a system perpetuates itself, but what are the reasons why patriarchy evolved in the first place? Psychological analysis has itself been part of the patriarchal knowledge disseminated by males. Freud, for example, based much of his work around the study of 'neurotic' women, and the idea of woman as the 'other'. Women were seen from the male perspective (What other perspective is there in a patriarchal society?) and thus deemed to be inferior. Much of Freud's work centres around the idea of penis envy to explain the process of identification that he believed girls experienced – the Electra Complex. According to Freud, a girl believes that she once had a penis, but that it was cut off by her mother as a punishment for something she had done in the past. By associating with her father, the girl's unconscious urge to have a penis is satisfied, and the envy of the penis diminishes. However, by identifying so closely with her father, the girl experiences anxieties about her relationship with her mother. Consequently, the girl represses feelings towards her father and then identifies with her mother, learning to think, act and feel in similar ways to other same sex people. It would be difficult to conceive a more male-orientated theory than that all females really wish they could be males, or that the male genital organ is so desirable, and this is a prime example of what Dale Spender refers to as the patriarchal belief that the male experience is the sum total of human experience (1982). Much of Freud's work is now not taken seriously, but this particular concept of penis envy has spawned an interesting alternative psychological explanation for men's desire to dominate – the idea of womb envy.

This concept attempts to explain the reason behind the entire system of patriarchy and male domination (Chodorow, 1978). The theory of womb envy is that the act of reproduction, of being able to bear and rear children, is such an overwhelming display of power and omnipotence, and one which men can never, ever have, that men seek to be powerful in every other possible situation.

> *Power of this kind, concentrated in one sex and exerted at the outset over both, is far too potent and dangerous a force to be allowed free sway in adult life.* (Dinnerstein, 1987:161)

Also, in order to play down their feelings of inadequacy, the role of motherhood is devalued, given little status. Jobs that are associated with mothering roles are also often given lower status (and thus pay) than other jobs. Consider teaching, for example, where the older the age of the pupils taught, the higher the status and pay is received. Indeed, there are very few male nursery and infant teachers; such work is often condemned as being concerned with wiping noses and tying shoelaces, rather than the immensely skilled professional expertise that is required to teach literacy and numeracy skills and also to socialise our children. Nursing too, is still completely dominated by women, although the fewer number of males in the profession manage to achieve the top jobs more regularly. The term 'male nurse' is still common. What is the relevance of such a term? Is it supposed to signify a distancing from female nurses? If so, why? Are male nurses performing a more important role than female nurses?

Radical feminism focuses on patriarchy to explain the way in which women are marginalised in all spheres of life and in all societies. Perhaps the major weakness of this theory, however, is that it assumes that all women have the same experiences and are equally oppressed. As we saw from the discussion of black feminism, women are not an homogenous group, inequalities vary between women themselves, between women in different historical periods and also between women and men. Not all women are controlled by all men.

Feminist theories have been developed as a different way of analysing the structure of society; to uncover what is going on from a female perspective, so that inequalities can be challenged and changed. All feminist theories provide different perspectives that may be more or less appropriate to different groups of women. All the theories contribute to a broader understanding of our society and hence to a more cohesive, inclusive structure that acknowledges and values everyone's experience, regardless of gender.

Theoretical explanations of the relationships between women and men help us to focus on the actual nature of society. Can there be a theoretical framework from which to explain the actual violence that appears to play a large part in many of these relationships? Violence represents the unacceptable face of male power over women. For some writers, violence signifies the actual failure of that power. Jan Horsfall, for example (1991:16), suggests that family violence is an indication that patriarchal relations:

are under duress either from outside or within the family.

She believes that battering shows there is a resistance to patriarchal structures, and if women accepted male domination unquestioningly, men would not need to resort to their superior physical power. Such an all-embracing theory, however, is rather patronising to those (many) women who are not in abusive relationships, and to those males who are non-violent, as it suggests that these women in particular have accepted and acquiesced to a patriarchal domination and it is only this acceptance of subordination which keeps them safe.

A continuum of male violence?

Some feminist writers (Hart, 1986; Kelly, 1986) have suggested that there is a continuum of male violence, and that battering or even murder of a partner is at the extreme of a scale that starts with something like wolf-whistling. From this view, the portrayal of women in the media, the sale of pornography, the constant display of women in sexualised positions on billboards, in newspapers, even in some places of work, are all types of abuse of a greater or lesser severity according to opinion. Accordingly, this perspective would regard all men as abusers, by using the definition of abuse as given by the survivors of violence. Abusive men often seek to define abusive behaviour for themselves and thereby frequently deny that their actions are abusive, although they may be differently understood by their partners. Jukes (1993:295) has produced a list of characteristics of the continuum of abusive male behaviour, which has been based on part of the Emerge counselling programme in Boston, Massachusetts. This list has itself been compiled by survivors of abuse from partners.

- *Physical abuse*, slap, punch, grab, kick, choke, push, restrain, pull hair, pinch, bite, rape, use force, threats or coercion to obtain sex or indulge in sexual practices which she does not want.

- *Use of weapons*, throwing things, keeping weapons around that frighten her.

- *Abuse of furniture, pets, destroying her possessions*, tearing or spoiling her clothing.

- *Intimidation,* standing in the doorway during arguments, angry or threatening gestures, use of your size to intimidate, standing over her, driving recklessly, uninvited touching, covering her mouth to stop her talking.

- *Threats of violence,* verbal or non-verbal, direct or indirect, self-inflicted injury – for example, hitting your head on walls or threatening suicide.

- *Harassment,* for example, uninvited visits or calls, following her, checking up on her, not leaving when asked.

- *Psychological and emotional abuse*

- *Isolation,* preventing or making it hard for her to see or talk to her friends, relatives and others. Making derogatory comments about her friends.

- *Yelling,* swearing, being coarse, raising your voice, using angry expressions or gestures, embarrassing her.

- *Criticism,* name calling, swearing, mocking, put-downs, ridicule, accusations, blaming, humiliating. Angrily waking her up from sleep.

- *Pressure tactics,* pushing her to make decisions or hurry up, walking in front of her, using guilt, sulking, threats of withholding financial support, manipulating the children.

- *Interrupting,* changing the subject, not listening or responding, picking up the newspaper when she wants to talk, twisting her words.

- *Economic harassment,* getting angry with her about 'where the money goes', not allowing access to money, the car or other resources, sabotaging her attempts to work, believing you are the provider and thinking that she could not survive without you, saying that the money you earn is yours.

- Claiming the *right to define* what is logical, rational, reasonable or fair in the relationship. Calling her stupid or otherwise defining her behaviour as illogical, unreasonable, irrational and so on.

- *Using pornography,* including home videos, against her wishes.

- *Feeling stressed and tense*, and using this to get into a frame of mind where you blame her for everything that goes wrong: things you can't find, mess, and so on.

- *Telling her* that if she doesn't like it she knows what she can do – pack, leave, and so on.

- *Not acknowledging* that the relationship is important to you, telling her that you don't need her or love her, and so on.

Many readers may not accept that all the factors mentioned on the above list do actually constitute abuse, or that women are as oppressed as a group as it seems to suggest. Jukes (1993) suggests that sceptical men (and women) actively become aware of all the situations in which women are put down by men, either implicitly or explicitly. Apart from the sexual stereotyping in the media, women are the butt of endless jokes that imply both their inferiority, and also refer to the degree of sexual attractiveness that they possess. Jukes suggests observing the pattern of behaviour of one's friends in order to fully appreciate the depth of sexism, or the assumption of male superiority over women. Areas of interest are control of the family car, the ability to spend money without consultation, control over television viewing, making tea for the children, and rooms or spaces that are solely for use by men (for example, studies, sheds, and so on). Acceptance of this 'natural order of things' is part of the process of socialisation and it is this endemic sexism that forms the basis of the continuum concept.

The concept of a continuum may be problematic; many women and men would regard wolf-whistling, for example, as a harmless activity carried out by both sexes, which merely shows appreciation of another's physical attributes. Many believe that to regard all male–female interaction as on a continuum of behaviour leading to violence may be both inaccurate and offensive, and serve no real purpose in the fight against patriarchal domination.

However, the idea of such a continuum may usefully place the responsibility for violent behaviour on the male perpetrators, rather than suggest that there is some complicity between men and women in abusive relationships. The view that violence in relationships is a shared responsibility is a widely established belief. Indeed, the notorious Judge

Pickles showed clear evidence of this in 1990, when, in a court case where a wife was accusing her husband of battery, he asked the woman:

How do I know you didn't deserve it?

Apart from the mainly male judicial attitudes, there is also evidence of the belief that women have contributed to their victim status in the field of therapy. Some practitioners believe that couples are dysfunctional rather than individuals, and therefore place responsibility on both partners to change their behaviours.

As Jukes (1993) observes in his book detailing his work with abusive men:

(The woman) is in a double bind. If she pushes towards him, he pulls away or abuses her more actively. If she withdraws, she resigns herself to not getting the intimacy and support she longs for. It feels as if she cannot win.

And this is precisely how the man is structuring the situation: as a competitive win/lose battle for control. She finds this bewildering; he can experience loss of control as terrifying. Traditionally, marital therapists have focused on the woman's pursuing behaviour, suggesting to her, for example, that she might consider giving her husband more space. As Jukes (1993: 271) notes:

I can readily acknowledge that he is unlikely to attend for any form of treatment if he is seen as being to blame for the marital difficulties, but is blaming the woman ... a better strategy?

Can feminism provide the answer to violence against women?

We have seen that there is no single feminist perspective, but what all feminist theories share is the belief that violence by men towards women must be referenced to the broader context of women's position in society, namely a subordinate one to men. Feminist approaches maintain that violence and, more importantly, the fear of violence controls the behaviour of women. The movement of women in public places shows a different relationship to the world than that held by men. Women are brought up to be aware of the possible dangers of being out alone after dark, and self-imposed curfews are often put in place when another woman has been raped in a nearby area. Thus women's freedom is severely restricted; they must remain at home, go out in a group of women, or put themselves in the care of another man. The freedom of men, one amongst whom is the perpetrator, remains unaffected.

Feminism since the 1970s has tried to give a voice to women, to make visible the victimisation of women. Since this time, women have increasingly reported violent and abusive men to the police, and they in turn, together with other agencies, have shown that they are more prepared to accept what women say. Feminists still believe, however, that the extent of violence is still massively under-reported. Also, the way in which it is regarded still suggests an individual solution for individual men is necessary, whereas feminism calls for an examination of the wider society, in which the social and economic subordination of women is addressed.

The power of the professional

What is a profession? Is midwifery one? If so, who benefits? The Collins dictionary definition of a profession is 'an occupation requiring special training in the liberal arts or sciences especially the three learned professions, law, theology or medicine'. Sociologists seek to clarify this definition by reference to three specific criteria: a unique knowledge base that takes a long time to acquire and to which access is limited; a strong commitment to clients' welfare; and the right to exercise a high degree of autonomy and control over its own work, usually by controlling recruitment and entry standards.

Many occupations, including nursing and midwifery, have actively sought recognition as professionals, not surprisingly, perhaps, as professions are seen as having a special place within society; they are better rewarded financially, they enjoy more control and they are awarded higher status than their non-professional counterparts. Professionals are deemed to serve the needs of society by being socialised, through an extended period of education and training, into an ethic of service. For the altruistic act of placing service to the community above self-interest, the rewards, both financial and prestigious, are supposedly high.

Nursing and midwifery has often been regarded as a semi-profession, because the education process involved has been deemed to be based on skills rather than knowledge, and what nurses learn in training is often believed to be ultimately determined by doctors. Also, the organisational control of the nurse's or midwife's role, what they actually do, has been thought to rest with doctors – the 'handmaid' theory.

In an attempt to free themselves of this perceived subordinate role, nursing theories and models have been developed that focus on the assessment and delivery of patient care, which clearly distinguishes nursing from its more clinical medical cousin. Midwifery, in particular, has built up a body of knowledge from midwifery research, which has affected practice. The vast knowledge that midwives have acquired about normal births, in particular, has generated a lot of changes to maternity care in recent years. An example of this can be seen in the great reduction of routine prenatal shaves and enemas and the drive to offer women greater continuity of carer, greater choice in childbirth and supposedly greater feelings of control. The aim in recent years has been to rid the profession of paternalism, and to offer more woman-centred care.

Part of the ongoing drive to professionalism has been seen as a way of gaining independence and status. Whilst this is completely understandable from the perspective of the skilled midwife who would like her (still mostly female!) extensive knowledge and experience acknowledged, how has the relationship with pregnant women been affected? Are midwives still 'with women'? Professions 'keep a body of specialist knowledge and control the consumer's construction of reality' (Kroll, 1996:181). The massive developments in technology have been said to depersonalise the experience of birth, particularly for the 98 per cent of British women who have hospital deliveries, despite lack of evidence that this is safer than home births (Campbell and MacFarlane, 1994). The reality of their situation is often influenced by the behaviour and attitudes of the midwives around them. Women, as mothers, often assume a grateful attitude that their baby has been delivered safely, when in fact, normal deliveries are 'the norm'. Actually asking patients or clients about the sort of service they want has been seen in the past, and is still seen by some midwives, as a threatening move likely to undermine the professional authority and judgement of those awarded the status of professionals. Yet research shows that women want intelligible information that will enable them to make sense of their situation (DoH, 1993). Identifying and meeting the needs articulated by women can improve both the outcome of the pregnancy and also the satisfaction of the women with the service offered. But woman-centred care, and establishing relationships of equals, are still seen as threatening by some midwives. The in-built fear of school teachers and members of the National Childbirth Trust who may well challenge the midwives' authority and power is well documented (Hunt and Symonds, 1995).

Has professionalism benefited pregnant women?

Has becoming a profession then, given midwives more status in the medical hierarchies generally, but at the expense of the women they seek to serve? Must professionalism lead to distancing from pregnant women? Clearly not, or if it appears to, the concept of professionalism needs redefining to allow it to encompass the thoughts and needs of those it is supposed to serve. Celia Davies (1995) suggests a 'new professionalism' that encompasses the way women communicate and exchange views by negotiation rather than assertion – the 'caring practitioner model of nursing practice' (Wilkinson and Miers, 1999:33).

So how can this 'new professionalism' be put into practice with pregnant women who may be experiencing abuse of any kind?

Midwives can gain knowledge and experience from the women in their care. Pregnancy and labour, although often following a similar pattern, are still individual processes experienced by individual women. If the feelings of individuals are listened to, and then shared with colleagues, the body of midwives' knowledge will be increased, and the 'seeing (of) women through the eyes of experts or through stereotypes' (Kroll, 1996:185) will be reduced. We have seen earlier how assumptions about those from different cultural backgrounds are often treated with suspicion or even dislike in society at large. Do such stereotypes persist in midwifery settings? Of course, not because midwives are inherently narrow minded, but because midwives are part of a society in which stereotypes and negative assumptions about people from minority cultures abound. Stereotypes get in the way of 'good' midwifery. The

Asian mother who seems to become hysterical during pregnancy may not have a low pain threshold or just be an hysterical personality.

As Tehmina Durrani relates in her book, *My Feudal Lord* (1996:185):

> *The nurses, unaware of my emotional state, scolded, 'Stop this nonsense, or we'll send you home'. The pains of labour melted into the accumulated agony of my absurd life, and I broke down completely. A collage of angry faces blurred in front of me as the hostile nurses chastised me for my hysteria … My hysteria had grown so wild that the physical agony of childbirth unleashed all the other pains of my life.*

The writer of this had in fact been subjected to violence of the most horrific kind over a number of years, as well as endless abuse and tormenting about her husband's affairs.

Midwives need to be open to individual women's stories, to find 'treasures buried entirely and hidden by techniques which assume that all people share the same common constructs' (Stainton Rogers, 1991). In simple terms, it means taking the time to listen to women and building on the relationship that should be formed when midwife and woman share a common and life-changing experience.

Pregnancy and childbirth should be a time of joy and exhilaration for women and their partners; but for some it clearly isn't. To be 'with women' midwives need to listen to their hopes and concerns, to engage in a dialogue which will enable them to communicate their fears about their domestic situation. In sharing their private feelings, women may find a midwife who wants to rescue them. This is, of course, a very understandable reaction when confronted with a vulnerable person – the desire to make things better is common to many of us. However, the perceived power of the midwife to 'sort things out', to simplistically assess a woman's situation and suggest solutions – seeing a solicitor, going to a refuge, leaving her partner and becoming a lone parent, with all the emotional and financial consequences, and so on, may in fact compound the woman's feelings of loss of control over her own life. Being advised of the 'best' option, may in fact lead to enormous feelings of guilt and inadequacy. Women in violent and abusive relationships know full well how damaging such situations are for themselves and their children; they need to be aware of what options they have and be given the space to think them through. Midwives can be genuinely 'with women' at such times, by using their professional power to inspire confidence, to empower the women in their care to take charge of their own situations. These issues are discussed in more detail in Chapter 6.

This chapter has explored some of the underlying causes of violence in our society, we have considered various models to explain the domination of some women by some men and we have considered the impact of academia on midwives and others in their interaction with women. In the next chapter, we explore the issue of domestic violence and childbirth.

Chapter 5

Domestic violence and childbirth

Yes, I've had black eyes, I didn't want to be pregnant, but I am and that's that.

He is always sorry, really sorry.

In this chapter, we will explore aspects of domestic violence and childbirth. We consider the reasons why domestic violence may begin or accelerate in pregnancy and examine the changing nature of violence in pregnancy. We consider the risk factors, the warning signs and the effects of abuse on the woman, mother and fetus and the baby.

We know that at least one in four women will experience domestic violence at some time in their lives, irrespective of their age, social class or ethnicity (Andrews and Brown, 1988; BMA, 1998; Mooney, 1993). These figures are likely to be under-estimated because many women will not willingly disclose abuse. There is still a widespread belief amongst abused women that domestic violence is still somehow their fault, that some inadequacy in their nature or action has led to the abuse; and, if it is their fault, it becomes something that they are ashamed of and are therefore unlikely to admit to or seek help or advice. Domestic violence is rarely an isolated event, it can start at any point in a relationship and is likely to increase in frequency and severity over time.

It is important to ask why should domestic violence be of concern to midwives? After all, pregnancy and childbirth are normal life events and for many women they provide an opportunity to reflect on their own health status and consider making positive health changes, like giving up smoking and eating a healthy diet. The majority of healthy women make contact with the health services and are motivated by a desire to improve their own health and the health of their unborn child. The media portrays pregnancy and childbirth as opportunities to nurture and protect the unborn child. The baby products industry feeds on the need to care, nurture and protect women and their vulnerable offspring. The advertising industry plays on images of men busy, proudly sharing the nest building; painting the nursery, fixing the less than perfect car, mopping the fevered brow and proudly supporting their partner in their joint achievement. The public perception is of a cosy, protective, nurturing time, where women are afforded extra privileges and respect; their condition is revered, their needs catered for and their peculiar dietary whims met. Pregnancy is seen as a time of expectation, excitement, extra special care, indulgence, love and affection. Pregnancy and childbirth are unique biological, psychological, and social events. Pregnancy changes a woman's body physically, her psychological needs will vary, but her experiences are embedded in the network of social relationships that surround her at this time. A woman's experiences during pregnancy, the care she receives from midwives and others will influence her future life experiences and the ways in which she will relate to others in the future.

However, in the midst of excitement, anticipation and pleasure is stress. The birth of a baby is a major life change; it changes relationships and patterns of life within families. It is a normal expected life experience yet still included in various stress rating scales, for example, Holmes and Rae (1967), as a stressful life event. The changes that pregnancy and childbirth bring are stressful for all women. The physical demands are significant, the psychological adjustments are considerable and the changes to the social networks within a family require major adjustments to be made. When the man is unsure of his role, insecure, threatened by the physical evidence that implies a permanent commitment to a woman and a relationship, or when either of the prospective parents have difficulty in adjusting to these changes the result is frequently overwhelming stress. For many women, perhaps as many as one in three, pregnancy is not the hoped for pensive, reflective nurturing time, but a time of increased threats and abuse and a time of accelerating, more aggressive, more life-threatening domestic violence.

Why domestic violence in pregnancy?

So why should a normal life event, albeit a stressful one, be associated with domestic violence? Stress is a well documented trigger of domestic violence, and pregnancy and childbirth are undoubtedly stressful events in the lives of both men and women. Part of the stress undoubtedly comes from the conflict between the unrealistic expectations of parenthood and the demanding reality where the rewards take some time in coming. As we have explored earlier in this book, domestic violence is much more than hurting someone physically and psychologically. Through violence, the perpetrators exert power and seek to control those whom they assault. Through this control and aggression, vulnerable pregnant women are less able to defend themselves, less able to take evasive action and so are more likely to suffer serious adverse effects on themselves and their unborn child. The violence may be physical, sexual, emotional and psychological. The woman will be confused by the mixed messages she receives – from the media which tells her that because she is pregnant she is special, and the message from her partner who follows his escalating brutal attacks with fervent expressions of regret and promises of reform. This confusion, embarrassment and a distorted belief that in some way the woman is responsible will be competing with her in-built psychological need to nurture and protect her unborn child. Thus domestic violence exists in pregnancy and childbirth. Outrageous, unbelievable but, like the once hidden and denied abuse of children, true. To many women, abuse and assault are a reality amongst the cosy images of childbirth. It is important at the outset to re-emphasise that whatever explanations are offered, domestic violence is never justified whatever the circumstances. It is never a woman's fault and there can be no excuse.

Campbell *et al.* (1993) have proposed four different categories of domestic violence in pregnancy:

1. Jealousy towards the unborn child.

2. Anger towards the unborn child.

3. Violence, specific only to pregnancy.

4. 'Business as usual'.

It is not unreasonable to suggest that some men will be jealous of the time and energy that a woman devotes to her pregnancy and her newly born child, but the jealousy is also associated with the fact that the man is no longer the centre of her attention. Anger towards the unborn child may arise because the child has usurped his place in her affections, or because of fear of the demands that child may make on his time, income or freedom. Pregnancy-specific violence is difficult to explain but Gelles' work throws some light on this. Sadly 'business as usual' means that pregnancy has not offered the woman the protection that she thought it might.

Gelles (1987) suggests that sexual frustration can be the cause of violence, whilst Bohn (1990) argued that the perpetrator may subconsciously be trying to terminate the pregnancy, as a form of antenatal child abuse. Helton and Snodgrass (1987) argue that the explanation may be in the man's perception of the fetus as an intruder. The man is jealous of the fetus, this is expressed in violence towards the pregnant woman and, as such, is a form of fetal abuse. Gelles argues that sexual frustration stems from the misguided belief that sexual intercourse should not happen in pregnancy, consequently the man blames the fetus and re-exerts his control by violence. Gelles argues that it is the readjustments in the nature and structure of the family that cause additional stress, which manifests itself in domestic violence. Bradshaw's (1987) work takes a different slant. Rather than resenting or being jealous of the fetus, the man is actually jealous of the woman and her ability to do something he cannot. This jealousy, it is argued, manifests itself in violent abuse. Bradshaw argues that while a woman is pregnant and by definition dependent on a man, he exerts his power and control by emphasising her worthlessness and helplessness. Indeed the control is so attractive to some men that they refuse to use contraception in order that their wives may be permanently pregnant and subservient. In Chapter 3 we have discussed the theories of 'womb envy'. It is true that pregnancy and childbirth are unique to women; giving birth is simply one aspect of life that men cannot do. This, it is argued by some, leads to overwhelming frustration and anger with women and their power that it results in violence. Whatever the reason, women are the victims and suffer the physical and emotional consequences of abuse.

The incidence of domestic violence in pregnancy

The incidence of domestic violence in pregnancy is unknown. No one really knows how many miscarriages are a direct result of violence and no one can really be sure how often premature labour is caused by violence. Andrea's story (see Figure 5.1) is one of abuse within pregnancy.

According to Bohn (1990), most studies report a prevalence of abuse in pregnancy of approximately 50 per cent. It is likely that domestic violence is massively under-reported, but it is probably more common than pregnancy-induced hypertension or gestational diabetes (Mezey and Bewley, 1997). Both of these conditions are routinely screened for at each antenatal clinic visit. This makes domestic violence a major concern of midwives and other health care professionals. It is a major public health issue, which has been largely ignored. In my own unpublished research into the lives of childbearing women living in poverty, as many as one in three women have described how they have been subjected to domestic violence at some time in their pregnancy. Many women during a second or third in-depth interview will describe the injuries they have sustained in pregnancy and take the opportunity to share details of the similar experiences of their friends and relations (Hunt, 2000).

Most published research suggests that domestic violence may commence or escalate in pregnancy (Mezey, 1997). Andrews and Brown's (1988)

Andreas story

Amy is a community midwife in an urban area. Her case load is varied – some women live in a middle class housing estate, others in more deprived inner city areas. She has seen evidence of domestic violence in her practice, but until recently has felt that it was not her business to enquire into women's private lives. Andrea is part of Amy's case load. This is Andrea's sixth pregnancy, and she still does not have a living child. In the past she has had a termination of pregnancy, a stillbirth, and three miscarriages. Amy knows Andrea quite well. She has lived in the area for some six years and Amy has been involved in her care previously.

When Andrea had a stillbirth at 32 weeks, last year, it was Amy who cared for her in hospital and later at home. In this pregnancy, Andrea's GP has decided that a course of hormone injections would be useful in trying to prevent another miscarriage. Amy called to complete the booking information and to give Andrea another hormone injection. For once the work load on Amy's patch was quieter than usual and she decided to stay to have a longer talk with Andrea. Andrea's partner, Keith, had left to go to work. Andrea was tired and still feeling sick; as she lay on the sofa she explained that she was planning to give up her part-time job in the solicitor's office. She explained that Keith had insisted and was anxious that she stayed at home to rest. Andrea looked upset, she was worried and had been crying.

Amy completed the paper work and asked Andrea if she could examine her abdomen and perhaps try to hear the fetal heart. Andrea looked anxious and slowly pulled up her jumper to reveal part of her abdomen. She explained that the fading bruise on her left side had happened when she turned over in bed. The more recent injury in the shape of a sole of a boot was more difficult to explain. There was no fetal heart and Andrea started to cry as she explained that she had had some vaginal bleeding earlier that day. Andrea was admitted to hospital later that day and had a miscarriage.

It cannot be known how many of her pregnancies ended in miscarriage or stillbirth because of domestic violence. But until this visit no one had suspected that anything was wrong.

Figure 5.1 Andrea's story

study of working-class women in Islington reported that 25 per cent had been subjected to violence by their partner. Helton *et al.* (1987), using a questionnaire design, found that of 29 pregnant women attending an antenatal clinic, 23 per cent of women reported violence. In this study 8 per cent reported violence during pregnancy and another 15 per cent disclosed violence prior to pregnancy. Hillard (1985) found that 10.9 per cent of women attending an obstetric and gynaecology clinic reported abuse at some point in the past, and 3.9 per cent reported abuse in their current pregnancy. One in five of these women were still living with the abusive partner.

In an Australian study using an interview and self-report questionnaire, Webster *et al.* (1994) found that 22.9 per cent of women attending a pre-natal clinic reported a history of abuse. The proportion of women admitting to abuse rose over the duration of pregnancy to 8.9 per cent at 36 weeks. Medical treatment was sought for injuries related to domestic violence by 31 per cent of those who reported abuse during pregnancy. In the USA, Gelles (1974) studied 80 New Hampshire families, half of which had a known history of violence, whilst the other half had no known history. Twenty-five per cent of women in each group reported abuse during pregnancy. In a subsequent study, again by Gelles (1987), 23 per cent of women specifically reported domestic violence during pregnancy. Bohn's 1990 review of the American literature suggests the as many as one in fifty of all pregnant women will be abused during pregnancy. Again in the United States, Amaro *et al.* (1990) found that 7 per cent of women attending a prenatal clinic had experienced physical or sexual violence.

McFarlane *et al.* (1992) found the incidence of domestic violence in pregnancy was 17 per cent and that it was largely a continuation of existing patterns of violence. In this study women reported physical assaults, blows directed to the abdomen, rape and sexual violence.

Gielen *et al.* (1994) reports that women may be at greater risk of domestic violence in the postnatal period rather than the antenatal period. In this study there was a 19 per cent increase in frequency and severity of violence in the antenatal period but a 25 per cent increase in the postnatal period. Campbell *et al.* (1993) reports that 9.5 per cent of a sample of 79 women had been repeatedly sexually abused by their partner and 13.9 per cent had been raped. In Northern Ireland, a study of women resident in refuges found that 60 per cent experienced violence during their pregnancy (McWilliams and McKiernan, 1993). According to Bewley and Gibbs (2000), blows to the pregnant abdomen can cause the release of arachidonic fluid from the damaged tissues. This substance is a precursor of prostaglandins and it is this which can lead to uterine contractions, miscarriage and pre-term labour. Additionally, stress produces raised levels of adrenalin, the result of which is the diversion of blood away from the vital centres and placental perfusion.

Whatever the truth behind the various statistics, pregnant women and those with young children are more vulnerable to abuse than other groups. The fact that even one woman is abused in pregnancy is unacceptable. Midwives have a unique role and are in a very privileged position. The nature of pregnancy and the experience of childbirth provide midwives with the opportunity to develop a confidential therapeutic relationship with women. The midwife can be an accessible source of support and guidance to a woman and has failed if she denies the existence of violence or pretends it not her concern.

The changing nature of violence in pregnancy

Pregnancy may increase the risk of domestic violence, indeed it may be a time when violence actually begins (Gayford, 1978). Work by Stark *et al.* (1979), Hillard (1985), Helton and Snodgrass (1987) and Bohn (1990) has shown that the pattern of assault may alter in pregnancy. Blows to the abdomen, breasts, genitalia and multiple-site injuries are more common. Hillard's study suggests that 35 per cent of women experience an increase in domestic violence in pregnancy. In Walker's 1984 study, women reported abuse during all three trimesters, and in 1983 Bowker's subjects reported an average of 4.5 beatings during each pregnancy. McFarlane *et al.* (1992) and Helton *et al.* (1987) demonstrate that repeated episodes of violence during pregnancy are common. Two or more attacks were reported by 60 cent of 117 abused women, 79 per cent reported multiple-abuse injuries. According to Bohn, one-quarter to over half of all battered women are also sexually assaulted by their partners and the abuser may also prevent the woman from seeking health care for her injuries or antenatal care in her pregnancy.

Risk factors for domestic violence in pregnancy

The single most significant risk factor in any form of domestic violence is being female. However, a woman is at greatest risk of violence in pregnancy if there has been a serious level of violence previously, as we have seen pregnancy does not offer any measure of protection. In 1985, Hillard demonstrated that abused women are more likely to be divorced or separated and be of higher parity. Teenagers are more vulnerable than older women; this may be because teenagers are more likely to be pregnant and more likely to be financially dependent on men (see also Chapter 3). Abused women are also more likely to have had psychiatric problems, and have attempted suicide. Unsurprisingly, they are likely to smoke more and drink more (Mezey, 1997). But as we have stated earlier in this book, women who experience domestic violence may be of any age, from any background, or ethnic group. It is an extension of a patriarchal society and reflects the relative lack of power women have in their homes and in society at large. As we have demonstrated, pregnant women are not immune from domestic violence. It appears that they are even more vulnerable to men's possessiveness and jealousy, their unrealistic expectations, their belief in their right to 'correct women' and their need to maintain or exercise their position of authority over women (Dobash and Dobash, 1991).

Warning signs in the pregnancy history

What are the signs that should ring warning bells for midwives? It is very important that midwives are alert to the dangers of stereotyping. It is easy to assume that the woman who is poor, not too clean and perhaps not too articulate is automatically a victim of domestic violence. This would be a misjudgement. The warning signs are easy to list but complex to interpret. The midwife should use her eyes, her ears and her intuition. Simply checking off risk factors will not be helpful in alerting the midwife to abuse. More than ever, the midwife needs to take time to listen, make careful eye contact, appear to have all the time in the world, be in a safe place and think. The midwife needs to listen sensitively, look carefully and assemble in her mind an overall picture, and take her time. It is likely that isolated events and odd signs will be insufficient evidence on which to make a judgement.

The midwife should be alert to the woman who shows signs of depression, stress, anxiety disorders, panic attacks and depression. This may manifest itself in frequent calls, visits to the clinic with apparently trivial complaints, late cancellation of appointments, or simply by non-attendance at clinics. Teenagers are more likely to be abused than older women, although according to Parker *et al.* (1994) the abuse of older women is more severe.

The midwife may detect feelings of low self-esteem. A woman who is isolated from her neighbours, family and friends, weeps and expresses an inability to cope, might even be harming herself by burning or cutting her body. As we have seen, she is more likely to abuse drugs, alcohol or other substances and she may express suicidal thoughts. She may have missed a number of appointments and been labelled a 'defaulter'. When eventually she does come to the clinic, or the midwife gains access to her home, her partner may always be present. He answers the questions and even knows the date of her last period! He stays for the examinations and may act as her interpreter. When questioned, the woman often explains she does not have enough money to travel to the clinic and does have access to a telephone. She will avoid looking at the midwife, and will often stare at the floor or her hands. She is unlikely to disagree with her partner, or even speak and she will make light of any injuries on her body (DoH, 1997). She may complain of chronic pain, particularly pelvic pain and other vague symptoms. There may be a history of repeated miscarriage, termination of pregnancy, unwanted pregnancies, failed contraceptive use, previous low birth weight babies or even physical injuries from previous abuse. These may include perforated ear drum, fractures of nose, limbs, etc. There may be multiple bruises in various stages of healing, new and fading bruises and, as in child abuse, a history that is inconsistent with the injuries (Bohn, 1990). The abuse may have led to an increase in alcohol and/or drug abuse. She will not enthuse about the forthcoming birth; she will be slow to answer questions and slow to initiate conversation with the midwife. If she has not met the midwife before or had a chance to form a relationship with her over a period of time, the chances of disclosure are minimal.

Many midwives will see a lot of women in the course of their professional practice who have some or even all of these warning signs, some will be victims of domestic violence but many will not. The only way to find out is by asking direct questions. This is explored in the next chapter.

Mabel's story

Mabel had lived with Ken, on and off since she was 17. She had moved around the local area and had lived in a series of local authority flats and houses. This was her eighth pregnancy. She was 23 and she had previously had three miscarriages. Last year she had a stillbirth at 32 weeks. No cause had been found. The child appeared normal. Her remaining three children were aged 4, 3 and 6 months.

Mabel went to see her GP when she was about 18 weeks pregnant. She had missed the antenatal screening tests, but said that she didn't want anyone poking her around anyway. She had failed to attend the midwives' clinic at the health centre and the hospital booking clinic. Labelled as a 'defaulter', the community midwife arranged to call at her house. The address on the card was incorrect, but a neighbour advised that Mabel was now living with Ken and his brother at another local address.

When the midwife eventually met up with Mabel she was sitting curled up on the sofa in the living room. The children were at home and her partner and his brother were watching television. Mabel seemed pale. She looked depressed and anxious. She said she was sorry that the house was in a such a mess and offered the midwife some tea.

The midwife began to fill in the booking clinic form and confirmed the details of her date of birth, previous pregnancies and family history. She had known Mabel for some time and was familiar with her obstetric history. As she took Mabel's blood pressure she noticed some cut marks on her wrists. She asked how the injuries happened, but Mabel said it was nothing.

The midwife then asked to test her urine and Mabel left the room. Ken told the midwife that Mabel had had a lot of backache recently, and said that she was always complaining of something. His brother laughed.

Mabel returned and Ken turned away as the midwife tested the specimen of urine. The midwife explained that she would like to examine Mabel's abdomen. She said that she wanted to see if the baby was growing well and if the size matched the dates. Mabel looked anxious. Ken got up out of the chair and stood alongside her on the sofa. His brother looked away.

The children gathered around, looking expectantly. The midwife explained that she would try to hear the baby's heart beat with a sonic aid. Mabel lay down on the sofa, with a cushion under her head. She lifted her blouse and lowered her trousers to below her pregnant abdomen. Her abdomen was covered with bruises, some had faded but were still visible. There was a mark like a cigarette burn on her side.

The midwife palpated the abdomen but failed to find the fetal heart. The midwife said slowly and clearly: 'Have you been hurt in any way this pregnancy?' Mabel turned away. Ken said 'There is nothing wrong with her, she is just a moaner!'. Later that evening Mabel was admitted to the gynaecology ward with another miscarriage.

Figure 5.2 Mabel's story

Mabel's story (see Figure 5.2) is not uncommon, but often the events go unnoticed. Miscarriage is relatively common, so is frequently dismissed and rarely connected with domestic violence

The effects of abuse during pregnancy

Domestic violence in pregnancy has an adverse effect on both the woman and her unborn child. At worse it may result in the death of either or both. In the 1994-1996 *Confidential Enquiries into Maternal Deaths in the United Kingdom,* there are reports of six deaths of pregnant women who all were apparently murdered by their husband or male partners. McFarlane *et al.* (1996) and Webster *et al.* (1996) report that women who are battered are more likely to suffer from epilepsy. It is believed that head injuries and other blows subsequently lead to epilepsy. There is well-documented evidence of increased miscarriage (Andrews and Brown, 1988), termination of pregnancy, premature birth (McWilliams and McKiernan, 1993), low birth weight, fetal injury and stillbirth (Hilberman and Munson, 1978; Hillard, 1985; Webster *et al.*, 1996). Mooney (1993) demonstrated that abused women are three times more likely to miscarry than other women. Physical injuries to the live fetus include broken bones, stab wounds, and fetal death (Mezey and Bewley, 1997). Salzman (1990) reports placental separation, ante-partum haemorrhage (Kelly, 1988), fetal fractures and rupture of the uterus, liver or spleen. Edwards (1997) describes two cases in which pregnant women were stabbed and kicked. Not surprisingly the fetus died as a result. The Yale trauma study (Stark and Flitcraft, 1996) showed that victims of domestic violence were fifteen times more likely to abuse alcohol, nine times more likely to abuse drugs, three times more likely to be diagnosed as depressed or psychotic and five times more likely to attempt suicide. Sexual assault may include rape, hitting, kicking or mutilation of the breasts and genitals (Bowker, 1983). Sexual assault may also happen in the postnatal period. Women may also be prevented from receiving antenatal care or fail to seek early antenatal care. Violent sexual acts can produce physical injuries to the genital tract and subsequent genital infections (Schei and Bakketeig, 1989). Plichta (1992) has reviewed the literature for the effects of woman abuse on health care utilization and health status. In this paper it is reported that abuse results in serious physical injury and death; abused women have significantly worse physical and mental health status and are more likely to seek medical care for psychiatric disorders. Physical health effects are reported in a number of studies, with women significantly more likely to experience chronic pain. Plichta reports that the risk of suicide is much higher for abused than non-abused women, as is the increased risk of substance abuse. Other mental health problems include depression, panic attacks, phobia, anxiety, insomnia and emotional problems. Unsurprisingly, rape increases the risk of having mental health problems.

The physical effects are easy to list but the emotional and psychological effects are more difficult to define and describe. A woman who has been abused has to contend with her physical injuries, but she will also experience a range of negative emotions. As well as experiencing many other thoughts and feelings that prevent her from leaving the perpetrator, she may also feel betrayed, inadequate, angry, abused, violated, distraught, isolated and have a low self esteem. According to Heise *et al.* (1994) for many women, the mental stress and the living in fear creates a psychological stress that is worse than the physical effects of the beatings. Her children who are probably witnessing the abuse are likely to have emotional scars, physical illnesses, fear of abuse and injuries themselves.

Sutherland *et al.*, (1998), working in Michigan University, have studied the long-term effects of battering on women's health. In this study the effects of intimate violence on the physical and psychological health of women were examined over time. They measured changes in levels of physical and psychological abuse, injuries, physical health symptoms, anxiety, and depression on three occasions; the first was immediately following exit from a domestic violence programme and at follow-ups 8½ and 14½ months later. Their analysis showed a significant decline in abuse, physical health symptoms, anxiety and depression over time. Ongoing abuse was related to increased physical and psychological health problems. Physical symptoms were mediated through anxiety and depression. In simple terms being the victim of domestic violence makes women sick, mentally and physically.

After the birth of the baby

The risk of moderate to severe violence appears to be greatest in the post-partum period (Gielen *et al.*, 1994). This is not really surprising, as compared with the relative tranquillity of pregnancy the postpartum period is stressful for most parents. Lack of sleep, a baby that cries without explanation, decreased sexual activity, financial and emotional stress all contribute to the difficulties of the postpartum period. In 1994 Donna Stewart, in a comparatively small study, studied the incidence of postpartum abuse in women with a history of abuse during pregnancy. Twenty-seven women (90 per cent of the participants) in this study reported a total of 57 incidents of abuse in the 3 months after delivery. The mean (average) number of incidents was found to be significantly higher for the postpartum period than for the 3 months prior to conception. Sexual assault has significant implications in the postnatal period. In another study, by Stewart (1993), a survey was undertaken using self-report questionnaires of women attending pre-natal health care or admitted to hospital. The aim was to determine prevalence of abuse in late pregnancy but also to investigate health habits, psychological stress, and attitudes about fetal health. The questionnaire was completed by 548 women, 6.6 per cent reported abuse during the current pregnancy and 10.9 per cent before it. Of the women abused in pregnancy, 63.9 per cent reported an increase in abuse in pregnancy, 66.7 per cent had received medical treatment for abuse but only 2.8 per cent reported the abuse to the prenatal care provider.

The factors associated with physical abuse included 'social instability' defined as low age, unmarried status, low level of education, unemployment and unplanned pregnancy. The other factors were 'unhealthy life style', comprising poor diet, alcohol abuse, illicit drug use and emotional problems. The final factor was 'having physical health problems'. Unsurprisingly, abused women were significantly more emotionally distressed and they had little internal control over the health of their fetus. They believed that chance played the most important role.

This study confirms a great deal of what we know about domestic violence and pregnancy. It is easy to blame the victims and label abused women as low status, unhealthy and having health problems. It is not difficult to understand why abused women might have more unplanned pregnancies, use drugs, have emotional problems and feel as if they are not in control of their lives. A more sympathetic approach would be to recognise that it is far easier for women with independent means of support to escape violence and the detrimental health consequences of domestic violence.

Satin *et al.* (1992) studied 2404 puerperal women in order to determine the prevalence of sexual assault, to characterise pregnancy complications and report pregnancy outcomes of assault victims. The prevalence of sexual assault in this obstetric population was 5 per cent. Those women who had been raped had a higher incidence of sexually transmitted diseases, urinary tract infections or vaginitis, drug use as well as multiple hospitalizations during their pregnancy. This study, undertaken in Dallas Texas, concluded that sexual assault was more common in urban indigent obstetric populations. They noted more frequent pregnancy complications but normal pregnancy outcomes. All the participants in the study were interviewed in a private setting on a postpartum ward. They were asked: 'Has anyone ever pressured or forced you to have sexual contact? If so, before this pregnancy? During this pregnancy?' If the patient answered yes, then they were asked if they agreed to a more in-depth interview. The prevalence of sexual assault was higher than expected. The authors acknowledge the unknown effects of psychological trauma and suggest that sexual assault be addressed in the initial antenatal history. However, they fall into the trap of believing that only urban indigent populations are at risk.

McFarlane *et al.* (1996) specifically considered the effects of abuse on birth weight. In their study of 1203 African American, Hispanic and white women drawn from public prenatal clinics in Texas and Maryland they found that the prevalence of physical or sexual abuse during pregnancy was 6 per cent. They found that abused women began antenatal care during the third trimester with abuse preceding the late entry. They found that abuse was recurrent, with 60 per cent of the women reporting repeated episodes. More severe abuse was significantly correlated with lower infant birth weights for all three ethnic groups. Abuse during pregnancy was a significant risk for low birth weight as well as maternal low weight gain, infections, anaemia, smoking and the use of drugs and alcohol. Women who were abused delivered babies weighing 133 grams less than women who were not abused. Abused white women delivered infants with the greatest reduction in birth weight.

Webster *et al.* (1996), in a study of pregnancy outcome and health care use, followed 1014 women who had completed an abuse questionnaire during pregnancy. The purpose of this Australian study was to determine whether pregnancy and neonatal outcomes differed between abused and non-abused women. They found that abused women smoked more cigarettes, took more prescription drugs, were more likely to have epilepsy and asthma and they made use of social work services more often. There was a higher incidence of miscarriage, pregnancy terminations and neonatal death among the abused group. Although abused women delivered infants whose mean birth weights were 132 grams lower than those of non-abused women, the difference was not significant after adjustments were made. Mildly and moderately abused women were admitted to hospital more frequently during pregnancy. They conclude that domestic violence adds significantly to the cost of health care during pregnancy and is associated with poor maternal and fetal outcomes.

Dawn's story (see Figure 5.3) illustrates abuse following the birth of her daughter.

Dawn's story

Dawn had visited her GP many times since her marriage to Steve and on at least eight occasions during her pregnancy. She had been treated for thrush, trichomonas and urinary tract infections. She had sought advice on depression, but this was put down to the problems she was experiencing with her supervisor at work.

After a long and particularly difficult labour, her daughter Josephine was delivered by forceps. Whilst in hospital Dawn was very tired, weepy and complained of perineal pain. Her perineum was bruised and the sutures were very uncomfortable. Josephine was a restless baby and slept very little. Dawn had decided to change the brand of baby milk twice but with very little effect.

On her discharge home, Dawn was visited by the community midwife, whom she had met in the antenatal period. After careful assessment of baby Josephine, the community midwife turned to give Dawn some attention. It was clear she was very unhappy, very tired and emotionally distressed. She had been at home for twelve hours and was trying to cope with the demands of the baby, a very sore perineum, full painful breasts, Steve's sexual frustration and his moody unsupportive behaviour. The couple had no other help.

The community midwife spent some time talking about Dawn's pregnancy and labour and her physical symptoms. They talked about the adjustment to parenthood and the unrealistic images presented in the media. They talked about how Steve might be feeling and how Dawn could best help herself and deal with the difficulties she was experiencing. The midwife was kind and reassuring. She explained what was happening physically and emotionally to both Dawn and Josephine.

When the midwife examined Dawn she found that her perineum was not healing well, her sutures had been removed and she had been forced to have sexual intercourse against her will. The midwife gave some practical advice, advised warm baths and listened. She said that she was very sorry that this had happened. She told Dawn that she had known this sort of thing happen before and also told Dawn that it was not her fault. She held her hand and was kind but not judgmental. She told her that she had the telephone number of a support group and Women's Aid, but did not insist on leaving the information. She said goodbye, and told Dawn that she would call again the next day.

Figure 5.3 Dawn's story

Domestic violence is not a comfortable topic. Women will avoid discussing it and staff will be anxious about their ability to respond if it is raised. As such, the abuse of women is quietly swept under the carpet. Yet domestic violence affects women and their families far more frequently than anyone could imagine. Instead of conferring immunity, pregnancy, it seems, can lead to an increase in the frequency and severity of violence. Violence in pregnancy has long- and short-term adverse effects on both the fetus and the woman and as such it is a major public health issue. Throughout the book we have tried to uncover those factors that motivate some men to abuse their female partners. The perpetrators of violence appear to use the vulnerability of the pregnant woman to seek to control her and to assert their authority over her. Domestic violence is rarely an isolated event. It can start at any point in a relationship and is likely to increase in frequency and severity over time. This makes domestic violence a major concern of midwives and other health care professionals. Domestic violence is a major public health issue which, until recent times, has been largely ignored by those employed in the UK health service. However, midwives, health visitors and other health professionals are ideally placed to support women living in abusive relationships; pregnancy offers women an opportunity for free access to a midwife; it would be a great shame if midwives were unprepared or unable to accept this role. In the next chapter we will explore the ways in which midwives and others can help.

We have seen that violence in pregnancy is endemic and a major public health issue. We have considered the factors that impact on violence in pregnancy and have examined the consequences for both women and their children. In the next chapter we consider what, if anything, can be done.

Chapter 6

So what can be done? Nursing and midwifery interventions

He gets jealous I suppose. He doesn't mind if the midwives see me at home, but he hates me going up the hospital. He said that I shouldn't go until the marks had gone. I missed that baby blood test though. He came for the scan but it didn't help. He said if it was only that size I had no excuse to be so bloody lazy! I still feel sick when I cook his dinner though.

In this chapter we try to answer the question, 'So what can be done?'. Faced with the trauma and distress of violence nurses, midwives, health and social care professionals are often desperate to do something. We begin by asking why many women in the face of violence remain in the relationship. We then move on to consider how nurses and midwives can help. We examine the use of direct questions, screening tools and other guidelines and consider some practical steps that can be taken. We discuss documentation, dealing with evidence and discuss the factors that may prevent intervention. We consider sources of help for the midwife and explore the ways in which health professionals can respond.

One of the most distressing aspects of exploring the topic of domestic violence with midwives and others is the awful sense of powerlessness that midwives feel. As health care professionals, they are so used to fixing things, making things better and producing 'happy endings' that a common reaction is 'Well I would not stand for it' or 'Why does she put up with it?'. In coffee-room huddles, midwives express their anger and disgust; they agree that those injuries could not be the result of tripping or falling, but many still hold onto the belief that domestic violence is a private business, and nothing can be done. Midwives may wonder if today's case of premature labour followed rape or other physical abuse; they may ask themselves and their colleagues if that woman's antenatal perineal injury could have a physiological explanation. But it is only by understanding the complexity of domestic violence that midwives can move from anger and disgust to more positive interventions.

When midwives and others are first introduced to this topic their reactions are a mixture of incredulity, horror, disbelief, fear and anger. Almost invariably someone in the group or the meeting says: ' I would not put up with it. Why does she stay? Why should anyone put up with abuse?'. Some enthusiastic if mis-informed practitioners feel that it is their duty to direct and guide women into leaving straight away. One midwife even suggested that a woman who stays must be mentally ill and, as such, be enthusiastically persuaded or forced to take evasive action, by leaving the relationship. Domestic violence is far more complex than that and midwives like others have to learn that quick fix solutions will not work.

So why does she stay?

The American College of Nurse-Midwives, in their pack *No Woman Deserves to Hurt,* explore the barriers to leaving (Paluzzi and Slattery, 1996:33). They use the following 'F words' to explore this issue: fear, financial, family, failure, faith, father, face, full, fantasy, fix, familiarity, and fatigue. Although this text is written for an American readership, the principles are applicable this side of the Atlantic. In the UK many women will be too afraid to leave; fear of the unknown and fear of change, even if the change might be for the better, cause women to resist change. The risk of injury and death is greatest around the time a woman tries to leave. Moving out of a marital home will have financial implications for the majority of women. The patriarchal nature of society means that most women are financially dependent on men. The cost of setting up a separate household will be beyond the reach of most women and the majority of women who leave their partners will experience a lower standard of living. A woman who makes the decision to leave will have to face the scorn and disdain of his and possibly her family. Men who abuse their wives are often very good at keeping up appearances; to others outside the relationship things may seem to be well. Those outside the immediate family will often blame the woman and hold her responsible for the breakdown of the relationship. She may lose more than her partner or husband; she may be separated from her friends and support networks. It is inevitable that women who leave will feel a sense of failure. As a woman she may believe that she should have been able to prevent the abuse. The family may share certain religious beliefs or faith that suggest that the family must stay together at all costs and this combined with a belief that children are better off with a father who abuses his wife than no father at all may make some women stay. Some women are part of a culture or public face that accepts abuse. One of the authors was once told: 'You see round here, men believe they have a right to correct their wives. If I get a beating, it's usually because I deserve it, you know I've nagged too much or asked for something.'

Having made the decision to leave, some women may find that the Women's Aid shelter in that area is full. She may be offered accommodation in another part of the UK, far away from any family or supportive friends. Faced with this option, she may slip back into the fantasy phase and believe her husband when he says that he will change. She may even believe that somehow he is capable of returning to the person she knew on her honeymoon. Strengthened by this fantasy she may resolve to fix things. She will be sure that if she tries harder, treads more carefully then he will really change and the abuse will end. When all this fails and she is abused again, she may lose the ability to believe that things can change. Faced with the daily familiarity of abuse she cannot see another way of living. Finally, as the abuse continues to take its toll on her health and strength, she is too tired, emotionally and physically just too fatigued, to find the energy to leave the relationship (Paluzzi and Slattery, 1996).

Domestic violence: a case for midwifery intervention?

Midwives are in a unique position to offer support to women facing this kind of stress and abuse. During pregnancy they have the opportunity to spend time with women, to listen to what they have to say and to listen to what they don't say. The therapeutic relationship that can be developed, especially when midwives are working in small teams or 'one to one' schemes, allows midwives the opportunity to ask more difficult and more intimate questions. For midwives who know the women in their case load, and for those who can establish some kind of therapeutic relationship, the opportunity will be there. As midwives, they can legitimately spend time alone with women, listen to their concerns and legitimately undertake physical examinations, both carefully and sensitively.

The systems for dealing with child abuse are well documented and despite some very public failures in the system, these procedures are well thought through and involve teamwork and co-operation between a range of professionals. Social workers, midwives, health visitors, district nurses and voluntary organisations and charities work together to protect children. However, in the UK there is no similar systematic approach to the detection of domestic violence, which is nearly always the abuse of women, and any intervention first depends on detection.

We know from earlier chapters that pregnant women may present with a range of physical and emotional symptoms of abuse. The midwife may learn by talking to the woman or by reading her notes that she has a history of frequent miscarriage, termination of pregnancy, previous stillbirth or stillbirths, premature labour, intrauterine growth retardation, smoking, alcohol or substance abuse; and the midwife may read that this pregnancy was unplanned or unwanted. The woman may have had admissions with urinary infections, pelvic pain, chronic generalised pain, and injuries of various ages, where the explanation does not match the injury. She may show signs of anxiety, depression, isolation and an inability to cope. Perhaps she is taking tranquillisers or analgesics.

The astute midwife will link these physical signs to a pattern of behaviour. The woman may appear frightened and excessively anxious, yet she will have missed appointments or forgotten to take treatments. She will explain that she cannot get to the clinic, perhaps because she has no transport or no money. When she does come to the clinic her partner will stay with her all the time, answering questions, taking charge and occasionally taking the opportunity to belittle her, make fun of her, or mock her pregnant state. The RCM (1997) Guidelines explain that the woman in this situation may appear frightened, ashamed, evasive, embarrassed and unresponsive. At this stage, it would be easy for the midwife to create distance between herself and the woman. Her instincts will tell her that there is something wrong, but in a busy clinic and without clear guidelines, adequate professional education and the back up of her midwifery and medical team, it is easy for the midwife to retreat to the safety of the booking form. Filling in forms and computer data are far more simple than asking direct questions. For many midwives, their suspicions will stay as thoughts without action. Many will simply not know what to do, or how to do it. The literature is conflicting – some argue that asking direct questions is outside the midwife's sphere of responsibility. Others argue that the midwife should not seek information that she cannot deal with, indeed asking may do more harm than good (Cochrane, 1997). We believe that the midwife must intervene and the benefits outweigh the costs. For many years, child abuse was ignored and treated as a private matter within families. Now it is universally abhorred and everyone would act to intervene if a child was at risk. We believe that this is the moment when the midwife must remember that domestic violence is morally and socially unacceptable and a major public health issue. It is also worth remembering that as domestic violence is so common and the majority of midwives are female, it is likely that many of them will have been subjected to domestic violence in their own lives. Women in all walks of life should demonstrate that they will not tolerate abuse against women.

The use of direct questions, screening tools and assessment guides

There appears to be considerable controversy in the literature as to the appropriate use of screening lists and the asking of direct questions. Much of the literature is American in origin, where it can be argued that asking direct questions is more culturally acceptable. Some writers, for example Hehir (1998) and Kent (1987), feel quite strongly that midwives should not 'snoop' for signs of domestic abuse. Indeed, in so doing they are abusing their privileged position. A similar attitude to child abuse was commonplace for many years, but as children were murdered or injured the sense of outrage became stronger than the 'British' need to keep themselves to themselves. The effects of domestic violence in pregnancy are so severe as to totally justify this type of intervention. We do not believe that midwives risk offending anyone, since women for whom this is not an issue will answer directly and the interview can move on.

Covington *et al.* (1997) sought to discover if using a systematic assessment protocol could increase the reporting of domestic violence among pregnant adolescent women, as compared with routine prenatal assessment. The study undertaken in North Carolina used a protocol to assess violence at three points during pregnancy. They asked only one direct question: 'Have you been hit, slapped, kicked or hurt during this pregnancy?' The use of this systematic assessment resulted in an increase in reported violence from 5.4 per cent to 16.2 per cent. The 'maternity care co-ordinators' (possibly midwives by another name) listed five factors related to increased reporting. These were: the use of a written protocol, asking direct questions, not labelling the victim, not naming the perpetrator and conducting multiple assessments. Their conclusions are justified; multiple, direct systematic assessments throughout prenatal care resulted in increased reporting of prenatal violence amongst adolescents, as compared to single, routine, non-structured assessments.

Gazmararian *et al.* (1996), in another North American review of the available literature, have consistently shown that when adequately trained, thoughtful sensitive health carers are taught to ask direct questions, the disclosure of domestic violence increases. The reviewers advocate further research to develop and use standard methods of abuse assessment. They recommend measures that include severity of injuries, and the period of time over which the abuse occurs. They argue that because violence is so prevalent during pregnancy and the effects are so detrimental, every woman presenting for antenatal care should be screened. The training of interviewers or assessors would need to be extensive to be effective. This of course has cost implications for any UK maternity service.

The Royal College of Midwives suggest the following initial questions:

– Is everything all right at home? How are you feeling?

– Are you getting the support you need at home?

The London Borough of Camden's *Guidelines for Health Professionals* version is more specific:

> *I don't know if this is a problem for you, but many women I see as patients are dealing with abusive relationships. Some are too afraid or uncomfortable to bring it up themselves, so I have started asking about it routinely. Is everything all right at home?*

Paluzzi and Slattery (1996) favour an even more direct approach: 'How do you and your partner resolve conflict?'

The RCOG suggestions for direct questions have been adopted and slightly modified by general practitioners, the Royal College of Midwives, accident and emergency room nurses, district nurses and many others. At St George's Hospital in London, a research midwife (Alison Howarth) and a research psychologist (Loraine J Bacchus) are currently (2000) involved in a project to investigate domestic violence in pregnancy. They are working on a training pack which includes questions that midwives can ask women. In the RCOG publication *Violence Against Women* (Bewley *et al.*,1997) the consensus of opinion is that the following questions, or forms of these questions, should be asked of all women attending for health care:

– I notice that you have a number of bruises, scratches, burn marks on your body. How did they happen? Are you in a relationship in which you have been physically hurt or threatened by your partner?

– Do you ever feel afraid of your partner?

– Does your partner ever treat you badly, such as shout at you, call you names, push you around or threaten you?

- Have you been in a relationship where you have been hit, punched, or hurt in any way? Is that happening now?

- Has your partner ever destroyed things that you care about?

- Some women tell me that their partners are cruel, sometimes emotionally and sometimes physically hurting them. Is this happening to you?

- We all have arguments at home. What happens when you argue?

- Has your partner ever threatened or abused your children?

- Has your partner ever forced you to have sex when you didn't want to, or made you have sex in a way that you were unhappy with?

- Has your partner ever prevented you leaving the house, seeing friends, getting a job or continuing your education?

- Does you partner get jealous? How does he act then?

- Does your partner use drugs /alcohol? How does that make him act?

Clearly these are difficult, sensitive and searching questions. They need to be asked in complete privacy without fear of interruptions or the presence of the abusive partner. The majority of midwives would need the opportunity to practice asking these questions in a safe place. Additional training, together with the opportunity to understand the social context of violence is essential. Nothing would be worse than for a midwife to use these complex and searching questions as a checklist. If this sensitive screening were to be seen as a task to be completed, a form to be filled in, with details alongside the date of the last period, name of GP, and so on, it may result in a mechanistic and uncaring input into a computer. The midwife would have her attention focused on the screen and the keyboard, whilst the woman answers these closed questions with a single monosyllabic yes or no.

We believe that the simple question 'Have you been hit, slapped, or hurt in anyway in this pregnancy?' is the most appropriate question to ask all women. The midwife should use her professional judgement and her communication skills to consider follow-up questions. The guides provided by both the RCM and the RCOG are simply that – a guide. As such, they should not be slavishly followed and used in a mechanistic way.

So what can the midwife do?

First response

There are some very clear, practical and positive things that midwives and others can do. The first is probably to stop. It is so easy in a busy clinic or ward to become totally focused on the task, the jobs to be done, the next woman, the notes, the telephone and all the distractions that serve to prevent the midwife from being 'with woman'. So first, stop, look and listen carefully. Don't interrupt her. Wait until she has finished speaking and then tell her that you believe her. Next, you can tell her clearly that you are sorry, you empathise with her position and you believe that domestic violence is never a woman's fault. We believe that it is also worth saying: 'This is not your fault, this is not some problem with you or the way in which you relate to your partner'. It may help to say: 'We know that as many as one woman in every four will experience domestic violence in her life; we also know that pregnancy can be a trigger for violence against women'. Don't make a judgement. Don't tell her to leave him. Don't say you would not stand for it. Don't hand her the telephone number of Women's Aid and shout 'next!'. Don't re frame her problem as an obstetric issue or a mental health problem. Acknowledge exactly the cause of her problem. Women are entitled to be supported, acknowledged and helped.

And next?

There are so many things that a midwife can do; it is so easy to take charge, call the police, ring social services, ring the housing department and contact the local refuge. The most difficult thing is to do nothing. Midwives must avoid becoming the knight in shining armour, riding in to solve the problem. What is needed most is a private, quiet, discussion where the midwife explores with the woman the choices that are available to her. This needs time, peace and quiet away from the busy clinic to allow thoughtful sensitive discussion.

Understanding what is happening

Anne Davidson, an experienced, American counsellor and trainer in the field of domestic violence, has argued that many interventions focus on immediate action. She argues that nurses, midwives and others are anxious to encourage women to move away from danger (Davidson, 1998). She has developed the framework of stages of change originally developed by Professor James Prochaska. This model is widely used in the West Midlands area to teach midwives, health visitors and other health care workers about the processes involved in changing behaviour and action. Prochaska *et al.* (1993) describe the process of change as having various stages. Individuals move backwards and forwards around this cycle as they consider and modify aspects of their behaviour. Consider, for example, the decision to stop smoking. The stages are described as:

- Pre-contemplation

- Contemplation

- Preparation

- Action

- Maintenance.

In the example of giving up smoking individuals pass through the stages of pre-contemplation, when they do not consider giving up smoking; they may believe that they are immune from the destructive effects of tobacco. In the contemplation stage, they begin to think about the options, perhaps the health messages, and weigh up the benefits of stopping smoking. In the preparation stage they might buy some nicotine patches, visit a clinic, telephone a help-line and give away their cigarette supplies. Assuming the model is followed, and without regression by moving in an anti-clockwise direction, the action stage involves actually not smoking and perhaps taking up some diversionary activity like swimming or walking instead. The maintenance stage involves continuing to stop smoking.

Jody Brown, of the University of Rhode Island, has used this model (Brown, 1996) to help midwives and others understand the process of change in abused women. She explains how at the pre-contemplative stage of change, women have a distorted view of their relationship with their abuser. She describes how they might lie to cover things up, believe they are responsible for the abuse, be accepting of violence, be unaware that any other options are available to them, believe that most people's relationships are like theirs, believe that they are totally dependent on the relationship for their survival, be reactive, be accepting, be isolated, but be hopeful that their partner will change. She has used women's own words to demonstrate their progress through the stages of change. At the contemplation stage, the woman acknowledges something is wrong; at the preparation stage she plans ways in which she might leave the relationship; and at the action stage she knows that a different life style is possible. This is a very useful model for abused women and for midwives and others to study. It helps midwives to understand why the twelve F's are barriers to leaving, and it helps midwives to avoid offering inappropriate and irrelevant advice. In order to intervene effectively, the midwife or nurse needs to have a good sense of where the woman considers she is in her relationship and experience. She needs to understand the events from the woman's perspective and know something of the woman's thoughts and feelings about her children.

Davidson (1998) has also used the Prochaska model to explain what is happening at the level of society. She argues that in the main, society is at the stage of pre-contemplation, or the stage before conscious thought or awareness. She believes that there is some illusion that we are more cognisant than we really are. But if there really was support for women experiencing violence, Davidson argues, then there would be 'an array of accessible resources in place and different laws for dealing with perpetrators'. Clearly there is still ignorance surrounding violence against women and a tolerance of something which many believe happens only to poor women or as a result of the abuse of drugs and alcohol. The myths that surround domestic violence are many and varied. Many people believe that women provoke violence because they enjoy it. This was the view expressed by Erin Pizzey in her early views on this topic. Others believe that because women will never leave their abusive partners, or if they do they will only return to the relationship when things have become quieter, any attempts at intervention are pointless. Davidson argues that the actions taken for individuals will always be limited whilst as a society we are in the pre-contemplative stage of addressing domestic violence. This view is probably depressingly true.

However, the midwife faced with the abused pregnant woman needs more assistance than a philosophical debate or an over-dose of pessimism about today's patriarchal society. The new *Midwives Rules and Code of Practice* (UKCC, 1998) in the section on responsibilities and sphere of practice states 'the needs of the mother and baby must be the primary focus of your [the midwife's] practice'. Domestic violence places both woman and child at significant risk; as such, the midwife cannot ignore it.

Return to action

Midwives must always work as a part of a team. When a woman reveals that she has been abused, this is the stage at which the inexperienced midwife must get help. The ward sister, the supervisor of midwives, the team leader, the midwifery manager, the obstetrician should all be able to offer the midwife the support she needs; but at this stage, perhaps, not all together. Every midwife needs another midwife with whom to discuss aspects of practice. It may well be a supervisor of midwives, but if she is not readily available then another midwife, whose judgement is trusted, should be available for a quick initial discussion. We have suggested that the midwife does not jump in and take over. We have aimed to explain through various models something of what might be happening. We have suggested finding a quiet, private place where the midwife can speak with the woman uninterrupted. But midwives are practical people and feel safer with a mental list, or even a few headings in a pocket note book, to guide their actions. What can she do? Her intervention may well depend on the stage the woman is at. Appropriate action will vary, but it is very important for the midwife to determine how dangerous the home situation is.

The midwife must be absolutely honest about the boundaries of the rules of confidentiality. If the midwife believes from what she has seen, or from what the woman has told her about the domestic scene, that a child is at risk, she is obligated to inform her supervisor of midwives and through her the social services department. This must be discussed with the woman at a very early stage in the meeting and the midwife must ensure that the woman understands exactly what will happen to this information. There can be no compromise in this instance. The requirements of the Children Act 1989 are very clear.

Safety planning and exit and escape plans

Sometimes very practical plans are helpful. The midwife or nurse can sit down quietly with the woman and draw up a plan. This often gives the woman some feelings of being just a little bit in control. The midwife can ask: 'Where have you gone before in order to feel safe?' She can give the woman the telephone numbers of the local and national Women's Aid organisations.

She must remember that these may pose an increased risk to the woman if her partner finds them. The midwife may give the names and contact numbers of others who will help – for example, local support groups, domestic violence forums, internet site details, counsellors, social workers, Relate, the Citizen's Advice Bureau, women-friendly legal firms and the Samaritans.

It can help some women to keep a diary (but probably only if she can find a private place to store it). In this they can record details of the frequency and severity of the violence. This may help them to begin to see the reality of the abuse. The midwife can ask if there are weapons in the house, and advise the woman against being alone with the abuser in rooms in which knives and tools are readily accessible. The midwife can discuss the benefits of teaching her children how to telephone 999 and ask for assistance and perhaps how to telephone a neighbour or friend in response to an agreed code word or signal. One woman had an arrangement with a neighbour that indicated if the porch light was left on during the day she was at risk. That simple arrangement led to the neighbour telephoning the police, who arrived as the woman's husband was about to stab her, whilst her two small children were watching.

It can feel a very positive action to pack an escape bag. This could be hidden with a neighbour or in a shed. The woman could consider packing a change of clothes for herself and her children, together with some money, spare car keys, medical cards and other essentials. It sometimes helps to have planned a place to go, by making an arrangement with a relative or friend. It sometimes helps to remind a woman that the labour ward of her local maternity hospital is open twenty-four hours a day, as is the nearest accident and emergency unit. She should always take her children with her. They are far less safe once she has made the decision to leave the family home and site of the violence.

Domestic violence is a very complex issue and midwives should never try to 'go it alone'. They must involve the supervisor of midwives, a team leader or other senior midwife manager at an early stage. It is likely that the woman will disclose domestic violence slowly and only when she is assured of the midwife's trust and confidence. Every maternity unit must have clear policies readily available that set out how the midwife should deal with referring a case of domestic violence.

Finally, if like Sophie (see Figure 6.1) as a midwife domestic violence is an issue in your life, remember that you need help too, before you can help anyone else.

Sophie's story

Sophie, a qualified midwife, was 26 and had been married to Peter for three years. Peter was a doctor and was currently doing a senior house officer job in plastic surgery. They both worked in the same district general hospital, Peter was well known for his sense of humour and his skill as a junior doctor. He had experienced some difficulty in finding work after his dermatology experience, and he did not want GP training. He believed that he could make a surgeon.

Sophie was pregnant with their first child and their family and friends were all very pleased. However, Sophie missed her last two appointments at the antenatal clinic. She managed to attend the next appointment and explained that pregnancy had 'numbed her brain' and that work was very busy. The midwife who had Sophie in her case load, met her and asked how everything was going with the pregnancy. Sophie described how she was tired and finding it difficult to cope with work. She looked sad and responded unenthusiastically to questions about her plans for the baby. The midwife noticed that Sophie was not as lively as usual but at this stage assumed that it was due to the combined pressures of work and pregnancy.

The midwife then noticed a fading bruise under Sophie's right eye, disguised with foundation. The midwife did not want to be seen to be prying but asked if 'everything was all right'. Sophie nodded but her eyes were cast downwards. The midwife was not quite sure what to do next. As she took Sophie's blood pressure, she asked about Peter. Sophie mumbled that he was well but was under a lot of pressure at work. The midwife realised that Sophie was not her usual self and said: 'Look Sophie, I don't know if this is a problem for you, but you know we see many women who are in abusive relationships. Some are afraid or too uncomfortable to bring it up. I always ask every woman I work with. Have you been slapped, hit or hurt in any way during this pregnancy?'

Sophie sighed, then began to get up to leave the room. She made a joke about how she knew how precious the time of a midwife was. The midwife

---

reassured Sophie that she had time to speak to her and in order to reiterate this turned away from the desk and the notes and faced Sophie. Sophie admitted that Peter did 'get a bit cross', but she was sure that it would not happen again. She explained that he was really sorry, and that he had promised it would never happen again. Peter had said that it was just an isolated incident, the result of the pressure and stress at work. If it 'got out' it might affect his chances of promotion. Sophie explained that Peter had brought her flowers and a teddy bear for the baby. She hoped the bruises on her head would fade quickly.

The midwife said that she was very sorry that such an event had occurred and that it did not mean that Sophie had done anything wrong. She also reminded Sophie how common domestic violence was and that it often started in pregnancy. The midwife then asked if Sophie would like to do anything that might prevent this happening again. Sophie said that she wanted to go home and that 'she loved Pete and trusted it wouldn't happen again'. The midwife smiled and offered to talk with Sophie again. They discussed how the midwife should record the incident and agreed that a separate record be held. They agreed a suitable time for the next appointment. Sophie seemed more relaxed by the end of the appointment and said that it felt good to talk about it.

Figure 6.1 Sophie's story

Documentation

The UKCC is the statutory body for nursing, midwifery and health visiting. As such, it has a legal responsibility to provide advice to registered practitioners on standards of professional practice. As an organisation it believes that record keeping is a fundamental part of professional practice. In its *1998 Guidelines for Records and Record Keeping* it offers clear advice on the content and style of records. These guidelines are equally applicable to records about abuse or suspected abuse. All records should be: factual, accurate, consistent, written as soon as possible after the event has occurred, written clearly with alterations or additions dated, timed and signed; jargon, abbreviations and meaningless phrases should be avoided, as should irrelevant speculative and offensive subjective statements. The UKCC (1998) advises that records should be written with the involvement of the woman, in terms that the woman can understand, be consecutive and identify problems that have arisen and the actions taken to rectify them. Above all, the records should provide clear evidence of the care planned, delivered and the information shared. These important principles under-pin the documentation of care when the midwife or nurse has to record information relating to domestic violence. Too often, records reflect routine responses and include meaningless phrases such as 'obstetrically well', or 'all care given'. There still seems a reluctance to accurately record what was actually said or agreed.

In many areas local Trusts have adopted a policy of hand-held midwifery records. It is vitally important that the midwife is aware that any thing she writes in the hand-held record is likely to be read by other members of the household and may place the woman at an increased risk. The midwife should discuss with her supervisor of midwives the preparation of a separate record in a confidential file that can be held in a safe place. The Access to Health Records Act 1990 gives patients and clients the right of access to manual health records about themselves. The Data Protection Act 1984 gives access to computer-held records. The UKCC (1998) advises that if a registered practitioner decides to withhold information from a patient or client (or simply not record details in her hand-held record) then they must justify and record this decision. The issue that is important is that domestic violence must be recorded and that the recording of it should not increase the danger to the woman or her family. We believe that it would be totally inappropriate to include a complex list of sensitive questions in the hand-held records.

- Seek and record the woman's clear consent to making a record, following her decision to disclose abuse.

- Explain why making a record may help her in the future, especially if the abuse leads to a criminal prosecution.

- The record should include any reference in her records to previous injuries or suggestions of abuse. For example, in July 1996, during her last pregnancy there was an entry that read 'injury to eyes, face and lip – Mrs Brown said that she had tripped on a loose carpet'.

- It is very important to write down exactly what happened and if possible details of other witnesses to the incident. For example, the record may read as follows: Date ... Time ... Mrs K Jones states that her husband George struck her on her head. This happened at her home address; the incident was witnessed by her two children, Steven and Mark Jones.

– Also include detailed descriptions of any injuries. For example, patient has bruising around her right eye. Her lip is cut, bleeding, requiring suturing.

– Include a description of the woman's psychological state and how she is feeling. For example, Mrs Jones was crying, she was upset and said: 'I did not think he would hit me but he did'.

– Avoid translating and interpreting the women's words. For example, 'patient alleges she was hit by her husband'. It is better to write: 'Mrs Jones states she was hit by her husband'.

– Avoid making judgements about the disclosure, or the injuries. Do not offer or record your view or opinion of the incident.

– Avoid any subjective data that could be used against the woman at a future date. For example, do not record: 'it was my fault, I always wind him up if I go on about him being late'.

– If you believe that the injuries are inconsistent with her explanation, say so. For example, 'the marks on her neck appeared to be rope burns, not a heat rash'.

– Record as accurately as possible the size, pattern, and description of the injury. Use a stick drawing or body map to indicate the location.

– Record any obvious damage to clothes or other personal possessions.

– Ask your supervisor of midwives or senior manager if you can seek the woman's permission to take photographs of the injuries. Most hospitals will have a medical photography department. The medical staff should be involved with this discussion and the decision. Document your plan and action.

– Photographs should be carefully labelled and stored in a safe place. They may be needed later by a court.

– Use the woman's own words to describe the incident and describe any damage to hair, teeth, belongings, clothing, and so on.

– Record in exact detail any medical, midwifery or nursing intervention, even if this is simply that the woman takes a bath or shower.

- Try to record the details of the assault. This may be difficult but is very important if the records are called to be used in evidence against the abuser.

- Record whether this incident is the first of its kind, or if similar assaults have happened previously.

- Do not state 'Mrs Brown refuses to leave Mr Brown'; this implies that any reasonable person would have followed your advice. Instead state 'After a full discussion, Mrs Brown chooses to stay at home'.

- Ask clearly and directly if the children have been involved in the abuse, remembering to explain the requirements of the Children Act 1989.

- Record your own impressions of the incident, including the woman's perception. For example, is she very protective of him? Does she think he will injure her seriously? Is she very frightened? Has she tried to leave the relationship? Is she isolated from friends, family, and sources of help?

- Keep the record in a safe place, separate from her hand-held maternity records.

- Ask the woman to read your notes and make corrections and alterations as she sees fit.

- Date it, time it, sign the record and include the names of other members of staff who have been involved, or who have offered assistance or advice.

Dealing with photographic evidence

According to the Department of Health website, midwives and others should explain to the woman that photographs will be useful as evidence if she decides to prosecute the abuser now or in the future. They suggest that the midwife should explain that the photograph will become part of the woman's medical record and, as such, it can only be released with her permission. Written consent should be obtained from the woman to obtain the photographs and a consent form should be signed. This should state: 'These photographs will only be released if and when the undersigned gives written permission to release the medical records'. A good Polaroid camera with colour film and flash bulbs is recommended, with the advice to take the photograph in a good light. An attempt should be made to take a close-up photograph of the injury, with an identifiable feature of the patient, such as her face or hands, to be included. A long shot followed by a close-up shot may be helpful. The photographer should sign and date the back of each photograph. The photographs should be placed in a sealed envelope and attached securely to the patient's records. Each envelope should be dated and marked 'Photograph of patient's injury'. The Department of Health also advises that as bruises are often more common two or three days after the injury, the patient should be advised to return at a later date for more photographs to be taken.

This may seem to be an over-complex response. In all cases, the woman must give her clear informed consent to being photographed. It is too easy to dismiss the process as being intrusive and possibly counter-productive, but any action that improves a woman's chance of stopping abuse must be taken. For generations, women did not report rape because of the complexities of the investigation process and the embarrassment of medical assessment. This plays into the hands of the perpetrator who continues to escape justice because someone believes that collecting evidence is too complex or intrusive.

Overall, the midwife must use her professional judgement to decide what is relevant and what should or should not be recorded. The UKCC advise that good record keeping is a mark of the skilled and safe practitioner.

Barriers to intervention

Bewley and Gibbs (1997), writing in the RCOG publication *Violence Against Women*, describe the role of the midwife in domestic violence. Bewley describes her experiences of running study days for midwives and her efforts in raising awareness of the issue of domestic violence in pregnancy. Through her study days and other experiences she has discovered that the issues for midwives were: lack of awareness; fear of making things worse and fear for their own personal safety; a lack of guidelines at local and national levels; fear of breaching confidentiality versus the possibility of child abuse; the pressure of work and economic constraints; and the lack of an interdisciplinary approach. Bewley argues that although these are valid concerns, they do not present insurmountable obstacles. But Bewley, like others who share her passionate concern about domestic violence, cannot solve the problem of a patriarchal society that is at the pre-contemplation stage of change.

Prevention of abuse of women?

Helton and Snodgrass (1987) argue that pregnancy presents a unique opportunity for midwives to observe and interact with pregnant couples. They believe that midwives can be instrumental in the prevention of battering, through education, research and advocacy. They suggest observing communication skills or the lack of them, and the ability to form support systems as couples interact. They believe that antenatal care may interrupt the cycle of violence at three levels – by primary, secondary and tertiary intervention. Primary intervention by education is achieved by including the topic of family violence at antenatal classes. Secondary intervention involves actively screening women for battering, early detection and crisis intervention for women and children, whilst tertiary intervention involves referring women to shelters, legal assistance and police departments. In this American paper the 'perinatal caregivers' can intercede in domestic violence of pregnant women by: assessing for battering as part of prenatal and postnatal care; providing community resources for battering; observing for injuries especially those with an inadequate explanation; using childbirth classes to observe parents' behaviour; and considering the safety of the woman first.

Currently the American culture and strategies for action in domestic violence are very different from the policies and schemes in place in the UK. Many will argue that the USA is far ahead of its British cousins. The health system is very different and the recommendations are not always easy to transfer to a British setting. However, by sifting and selecting, there are many useful models and practices for British health carers to follow.

Who can help the midwife?

As Bewley and Gibbs (1997) have so clearly demonstrated, coping with domestic violence is distressing and fearful for many midwives. As previously indicated, some midwives may be trying to face issues that are unresolved in their own lives. A midwife who is herself abused may have some difficulty in helping an abused pregnant woman who is part of her case load. The first source of help must be the supervisor of midwives. In many areas there are now more experienced midwives who have undertaken additional training to prepare them for this role. The supervisor should be wise, capable and have some idea about what to do and how to support the midwife faced with this issue. In other areas supervisors are still few and far between; some supervisors are sadly unapproachable and have not been able to separate their punitive disciplinary role from that of kind, supportive mentor. In many situations, clinical supervision can be the answer. There are a variety of models of clinical supervision, but the evidence suggests that its success depends to a large extent on the person providing the support. Butterworth and Faugier (1996) have demonstrated that the clinical supervisor should generate professional respect in terms of their experience, credibility, knowledge base, competency, accessibility and confidentiality – all the characteristics of a good supervisor of midwives. All midwives facing difficult clinical situations need the opportunity to explore the issues with a wise friend, whatever their title. They will also need to be reminded that they cannot solve every problem and should be realistic as to their goals.

Exploring professional responses

It is important to understand how influential the midwife and other health care professionals can be in a woman's experience of domestic violence. The Domestic Violence Project Inc. of Kenosha, Wisconsin, has developed the 'Medical Power and Control Wheel' model and 'The Empowerment Wheel' to illustrate some aspects of this complex relationship. Midwives can either be part of the woman's problem, exerting power and control, or they can be part of the solution by acting as the woman's advocate. If she is part of the problem, then she is bent on exerting her medical power and seeking always to control events. This can escalate the danger, put the woman at greater risk and in fact increase her entrapment. Each aspect interacts with other aspects, like the spokes in a wheel; each individual group of actions supports other actions (see Figure 6.2).

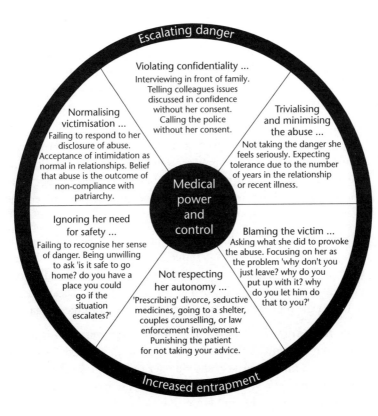

Figure 6.2 The Medical Power and Control Wheel

[The Medical Power and Control Wheel is based on the Power and Control and Equality Wheel, developed by the Domestic Abuse Intervention Project, Duluth, MN.]

She may do this by:

– *Violating confidentiality*. This might include chatting to colleagues about a woman in your care, not arranging to see the woman alone or in a private place or calling the police without her consent. It may mean inadvertently discussing a woman's circumstances in a relatively public place; the ward hand-over often takes place in the corridor or at the nurses station, where there is a constant through flow of people – doctors, domestics, pathology technicians all pass by. Midwives must remember that information should be exchanged and shared on a need-to-know basis. If a woman has found the courage to disclose abuse, the least she expects is the right to ensure that information remains private and confidential to those who need to know. Anything less than this means that midwives, in collusion with the medical staff, are exerting their power and control over a woman who has placed her trust in their hands.

- *Trivialising and minimising abuse.* Not taking her seriously, not believing what she says, expecting her to put up with it. Throwaway comments and asides that imply she should put up with the situation are unacceptable. Comments suggest that all men have weak points, or that she is somehow to blame, take power away from women and exert the control of the medical and midwifery staff.

- *Blaming her.* By asking what she did to prompt the attack, focusing on her as the problem. For example,'Why don't you just leave?' Comments that suggest that the woman is a hapless victim who is incapable of taking control of her life, all serve to accentuate the power of the professionals and diminish the power of the woman.

- *Not respecting her autonomy.* Respecting autonomy means respecting an individual's right to freedom, independence, and decision making. It means respecting her right to make choices even when as a midwife you think those choices are wrong. It means not telling her what to do, and criticising her when she fails to follow your advice. To be an advocate, the midwife has to be non-judgmental. She or he must recognise their own prejudices and accept the woman's strategy for dealing with her life, whether this involves action or non-action.

- *Ignoring her need for safety.* It is so easy to 'wash your hands' of someone who fails to follow your 'expert' advice. Many midwives may find that a woman's rejection of their advice leads to a disinterest in her problem. This is difficult to deal with but it requires the midwife to accept that her advice is not accepted. It then requires the midwife to pause and look again at how she might help. By not asking her 'Is it safe to go home?', the midwife has failed to recognise the woman's needs. It takes a special midwife to keep on supporting a woman who appears to reject all the advice she offers.

- *Normalising victimisation.* For many midwives the fact that domestic violence is an everyday feature of the lives of some pregnant women is too difficult to accept. If a woman discloses abuse and it is ignored by the midwife, control has again been seized by the midwife. The woman, weakened by abuse is further weakened by the midwife who either fails to respond to disclosure or says that it is not her business. Midwives who preach that abuse and intimidation are normal in relationships further serve to disempower the woman and enhance the power of the professional further.

So how might the midwife act as an advocate and empower the abused woman?

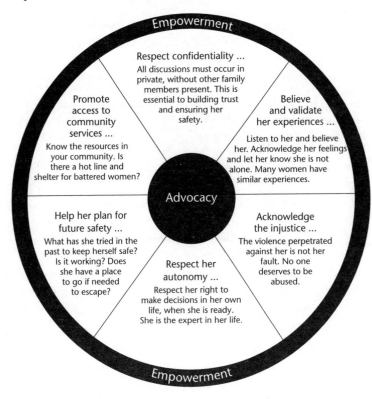

Figure 6.3 The Empowerment Wheel

[The Empowerment Wheel is based on the Power and Control and Equality Wheel, developed by the Domestic Abuse Intervention Project, Duluth, MN.]

The model shown in Figure 6.3 is also based on the idea of a wheel, each section interacting with other sections, strengthening and empowering women through advocacy. A midwife can support a woman in the following ways:

- *Respecting confidentiality.* The midwife must not only respect the woman's wishes but be seen to respect her privacy, her views, her wishes. The midwife must take care to arrange to talk to the woman without her partner or other members of the family present. She must acknowledge her right to refuse to undertake a particular course of action, even when that course of action seems sensible and logical to the midwife.

- *Believe and validate her experiences.* Midwives are very good at doing and find it more difficult to find the time to do nothing except listen. Acknowledging, supporting and caring can be satisfying actions for the midwife.

- *Acknowledge the injustice.* Midwives should be outraged about domestic violence, they should say clearly that it is not her fault and support her in her decisions.

- *Respect her autonomy.* Simply respect her right to make her own decisions, make plans and try solutions.

- *Help her plan for future safety.* Sometimes this means just talking and thinking. Helping a woman to explore her options is a vital part of the midwife's role in being 'with woman'. When a woman is hurt, humiliated, oppressed it is often difficult for her to remember the friends who have helped her out in the past. When her experience of domestic violence has left her frightened and ashamed it is difficult for her to be assertive and positive in planning her life. A midwife can be her friend and her advocate.

- *Promote access to the community services.* All midwives should know the telephone numbers of Women's Aid, the names of local 'woman-friendly' solicitors, the local number for social services, local domestic violence forums, the local police, perhaps also the local church and the Samaritans. Talking can really help.

Finally midwives themselves need help. Domestic violence must become a priority for NHS Trusts. Each Trust should have a clear policy and guidelines for asking questions and making referrals where appropriate. Midwives cannot deal with this major public health issue in isolation; a multi agency approach is essential.

This chapter has set out the practical ways in which midwives and other health and social care professionals can help women. It has also explored how midwives may need help themselves. It has recognised that for some women help is in the shape of a kind friend who supports her decision to stay in an abusive relationship. In the next chapter, we consider who else might be able to help women who are in violent relationships.

Chapter 7

Who else can help?

I know that some day I will have to leave him, that is if he has not killed me first. But what can I do? Here I am pregnant again, too late for an abortion. Anyway the doctor said that I should go for a test first, I missed the appointment then well ... he has been better this summer – the World Cup was on, then they were knocked out. It will be better later, when the baby is born, especially if it is a lad.

This chapter brings together the help that is offered by other agencies. It begins by exploring the role of the law and the changes in civil law that may be helpful to some women. It examines the Family Law Act and the use of various orders that may be put in place to protect women. We then consider the issues in relation to the Children Act and briefly the effects that domestic violence may have on some children. We examine the role of the police and consider the ways in which policing has changed to more sensitively reflect the needs of some women. We also examine how for some women calling the police may not be the answer. We consider the role of domestic violence units and the role of voluntary agencies such as Women's Aid. We briefly consider treatment for the abusers and the abused. Complex problems demand complex solutions and this chapter examines some of the ways in which some women can be helped.

The Family Law Act 1996

The first real change in the civil law relating to domestic violence came into operation in October 1997. The Family Law Act 1996 sets out a range of measures available to Family Courts. The Law Commission report, *Family Law, Domestic Violence and Occupation of the Family Home*, provides the background to the changes in legislation. The term violence is used in two senses. The first is the use, or threat of use, of physical force against a victim in the form of assault or battery. The report points out that in the context of the family, there is a wider meaning which extends abuse beyond physical assaults to include physical, sexual, psychological molestation or harassment. In fact, it now includes any action that has a serious detrimental effect upon the health and well-being of the victim, even if there is no physical force involved.

The Non-Molestation Order

Molestation covers a wide range of behaviour. It is more than physical violence and in order to obtain a Non-Molestation Order there has to be evidence of molestation. The range of 'non-violent' harassment or molestation behaviours include:

- Persistent pestering and intimidation through shouting, denigration, threats or argument.
- Nuisance telephone calls.

– Damaging property.

– Following the applicant about.

– Calling repeatedly at her home or place of work.

– Calling frequently and unexpectedly at unsocial hours when the victim is afraid.

– Installing a mistress into the marital home.

– Filling car locks with super glue.

– Writing anonymous letters.

– Pressing one's face against a window whilst brandishing papers.

(From the Law Commission Report, *Family Law, Domestic Violence and Occupation of the Family Home*.)

A Non-Molestation Order prohibits a person from molesting another person who is associated with him or her and prohibits a person from molesting a relevant child. The court can issue an order that restrains the respondent from 'assaulting, molesting, or otherwise interfering' with the applicant. The order may include a precise injunction against specific kinds of behaviour and may be for a specified duration or until a further order is made. It can be discharged by the court on application by the respondent or by the person who applied for the order.

Undertakings

An Undertaking is a promise by the respondent either to do, or not to do, some specific act and/or agreeing to leave the home. It is an alternative to the making of a court order. In simple terms it is a promise to the court. An Undertaking can be accepted from a party to proceedings in which a court would have the power to make an Occupation Order or a Non-Molestation Order. These orders are not acceptable where there is violence or a threat of violence. If both parties agree to an Undertaking the advantages are: firstly, the respondent makes no admission that any allegations are true and the court does not make any findings of fact in relation to the allegations; secondly, an Undertaking avoids the need for a contested hearing; thirdly, the applicant is given the same protection as he, or she, would have in a Non-Molestation Order or Occupation Order. However, although the sanctions for a breach of an Undertaking are the same as those of a breach of an order, no powers of arrest can be attached because an Undertaking in not an order of the court. An Undertaking may be given in writing in a court or to a solicitor acting on the respondent's behalf. A prescribed form is used. An Undertaking given to the court in proceedings under the Family Law Act 1996 is enforceable as if it were an order of the court. If the order is disobeyed the respondent can be fined £50 for every day that he is in default, or be committed to custody until he remedies the default. This, of course, assumes that the respondent has sufficient resources to pay the fine and is willing to do so.

Occupation Order

As part of the implementation of the Family Law Act 1996, courts were given powers to regulate the occupation of the family home. An Occupation Order is an order, enforceable against the respondent, giving a right to enter and/or remain in occupation of a dwelling house. This may be an order where a person has a legal right to occupy already, but where an order is in force it can be a punishable contempt for a respondent to fail to obey it, or seek to frustrate it. An order is normally only issued if there has been misconduct on the part of the respondent. This will usually involve proving the threat of unlawful violence or a sexual offence. Applicants for an Occupation Order may be a spouse or former spouse, co-habitants or former co-habitants who are entitled to occupy a home, and spouses/co-habitants who are not otherwise legally entitled to occupy. The court will decide whether to grant an application, the content and the duration of the order. There are five categories of applicant. These include:

– An applicant who already has a right to occupy and the order is made against 'any associate person' who is, or has been, sharing the home. Ancillary orders can be made, including provision for payment of rent or mortgage payments.

– A 'former spouse', when the respondent former spouse has a right to occupy.

– A former co-habitant who is entitled to occupy.

– A spouse or former spouse, when neither has a right to occupy.

– An applicant who is a co-habitant or former co-habitant and neither has a right to occupy.

Most women will need the help of a solicitor to clarify the meaning and significance of the terms 'associated persons', 'relevant child', 'significant harm' and 'matrimonial home rights'. 'Associated persons' include spouses, those who have been co-habitants, persons who have agreed to marry, persons who are living, or have lived in the same household, other than employees, tenants and lodgers. A 'relevant child' is a child living with, or who might reasonably be expected to live with, either party. The court must also consider whether the applicant or any relevant child is likely to suffer 'significant harm' attributable to the conduct of the respondent. 'Harm' is defined as ill-treatment or the impairment of health for an adult, and includes impairment of development for a child. Ill-treatment of a child is further defined and includes sexual abuse. The court must consider harm in the past and the threat of harm in the future. 'Matrimonial Home Rights' confer upon a spouse the same rights that the other spouse, who is entitled to occupy, has in relation to a dwelling-house. This means that in effect a woman who does not legally own a house can in fact apply for an Occupation Order against an associate person in the same way that a person with a right to occupy can.

These orders sound helpful and fair, but for a woman who is terrified, injured and fearful for the safety of her children they may seem unrealistic and out of reach.

Enforcement: remand and arrest

If a respondent is brought to a court following arrest under the power of arrest or under a warrant for arrest, the court may proceed to deal with the respondent immediately, or may remand him or her to appear before the court. Enforcement may be adjourned to enable the respondent to seek legal representation or to allow him or her the opportunity to produce evidence to deny the breach of the order. A remand may be in custody or on bail. Bail may be unconditional or subject to conditions. The court may also consider variation or discharge of an Occupation Order or Non-Molestation Order.

The court also has the power of arrest, designed to encourage compliance with a Non-Molestation Order or Occupation Order. The power of arrest must be attached to an Occupation Order where both parties have been given notice of a hearing and where it appears that there has been actual or threatened violence against the applicant or relevant child.

A power of arrest need not be attached to any order if the court is satisfied that despite the occurrence of violence, or the threat of it, the applicant or relevant child will be adequately protected by the making of the order itself. If there is no power of arrest attached to the order the applicant may apply to the court for the issue of a warrant for the respondent's arrest, whenever the applicant considers that the respondent has failed to comply with the order.

The interaction with the Children Act 1989

The Family Law Act 1996 has to be considered in its interaction with the Children Act 1989. This act places the emphasis upon the duties and responsibilities of the parent rather than on the rights of the parent. This applies even where the child is not living with the parent. One of the most important principles of the Children Act 1989 is that of safeguarding the welfare of the child. When a court determines any question in relation to the upbringing of a child, or the administration of a child's property and the income from it, the child's welfare will be the court's paramount consideration. The court must have regard to the principle that any delay in determining the question is likely to prejudice the welfare of the child. The court must take into account the wishes and feelings of the child, her and his physical and emotional needs, the likely effect on her/him of any change in circumstances, hers/his age, sex, background and any characteristics of hers/his which the court considers relevant. The court must also consider any harm which she/he has suffered or is at risk of suffering; how capable each of her/his parents, and other persons are at meeting her/his needs and the range of powers available to the court under the Act (Dimond, 1994:291). There are key areas where the interaction between the Children Act 1989 and the Family Law Act 1996 are important. These are the use of exclusion requirements, Undertakings, Emergency Protection Orders and Interim Care Orders. Both Occupation Orders and Non-Molestation Orders must be considered in the context of the Children Act 1989. Whenever a court makes an order, the paramount consideration must be the child's welfare. The effect of this may be to place the mother's needs in a subservient position.

The issue of child abuse, its detection and the subsequent actions that a midwife should take are complex and beyond the scope of this book. However, as children are those most likely to witness domestic violence their needs cannot be ignored. There is clear evidence of a relationship between domestic violence and child abuse. Connors *et al.* (1992:325) demonstrates that 'the lowest rates of child abuse are among parents who do not hit one another, with high violence-prone husbands and wives the most likely child abusers'. O'Hagan and Dillenburger (1995) argue that if hitting one another is part of the relationship pattern in a family, it does not have to reach crisis proportions to have negative effects. Many children are hit, smacked or slapped on a daily basis and this is still not considered to be abuse.

Dimond (1994: 292) states:

> *Where the midwife has reasonable cause to suspect that a child in the family of a client is being abused she must take appropriate action. To make the diagnosis is a weighty matter.*

As the guidelines on interagency co-operation state (Home Office DOH, DES, Welsh Office 1991):

> *the difficulties of assessing the risk of harm to a child should not be underestimated. It is imperative that everyone who deals with allegations and suspicions of abuse maintains an open and inquiring mind*

Other relevant legislation includes the Protection from Harassment Act 1997 and the Crime and Disorder Act 1998.

It could be argued that these orders tend to assume a logical, law abiding citizen who is in a minor degree of difficulty. The intrinsically sexist nature of the British judiciary system leaves many people somewhat cynical as to the benefits. Fines and short periods of imprisonment are unlikely to solve the problem of domestic violence. Imposing a fine may even aggravate the situation. Involving the law makes the violence a public matter not a private matter and for many women such action increases the risk of violence and even murder.

The police

Violence against women has only relatively recently been recognised as a problem by welfare and legal-enforcement agencies such as social services and the police. One of the major reasons for this lack of recognition has been the fact that statistics relating to marital violence are known to be wildly inaccurate, mainly due to the extent of under-reporting of such offences. A major study by Dobash and Dobash (1980) discovered that only 2 of 98 assaults were ever reported to the police, despite the fact that all 98 incidents involved relatively serious injuries and fell within the bounds of criminal offences. Later studies, Binney *et al.* (1981), *The Women's National Commission Report* (1985) and Horley (1988) confirm the trend of massive under-reporting, each suggesting that only 2 per cent of violent incidents are reported to the police, and that assault by males on their partners is the second most common form of violence that is actually reported. What statistics show then, is only the tip of the domestic violence iceberg; the vast majority of violent assaults remain part of the 'dark figure'. We shall now consider what influences are at work which make it likely that a woman will report a lost purse to the police but not a physical assault on her person by someone she can identify.

Horley (1988) shows that one of the main reasons given by the women in her study for not reporting violent incidents to the police, was that they did not feel that the police would be sympathetic to their individual circumstances. Over the past fifteen years, individual police forces have varied in their recognition of, and response to, marital violence. The purpose of this book is not to condemn the police across the board, but rather to acknowledge how services have been improved, and what still remains to be changed. Only by identifying both good and bad practices can the overall framework of response be improved, and battered women receive the service they desperately deserve.

The *Select Committee Report on Violence in Marriage* (1975) is testament to how far the police forces in Britain have changed their public attitudes. The following is an extract from the evidence presented by the Association of Chief Police Officers (as quoted in O'Donnell, 1988:366):

> *It is important to keep 'wife battering' in its correct perspective and realise that this loose term is applied to incidents ranging from a very minor domestic fracas where no police action is really justified, to the more serious incidents of assaults occasioning grievous bodily harm and unlawful woundings. Whilst such problems take up considerable police time during say, 12 months, in the majority of cases the role of the police is a negative one. We are, after all, dealing with persons 'bound in marriage', and it is important for a*

host of reasons to maintain the unity of the spouses.

This comment encapsulates an important principle that underpinned much of police intervention in marital disputes: that where violence took place between people with family ties, it could largely be regarded as a private, rather than as a public matter, and hence left to the individuals themselves to resolve. Of course, the issue we need to consider is whose privacy is being safeguarded? Certainly not the wife of a policeman whose local police officer and doctor both felt that she herself was a highly neurotic woman whose husband was, as a 'creative' person, given to volatile mood swings. Despite such mood changes, often resulting in serious violence, the local police did not regard this as a case for intervention, presumably because the couple were 'bound in marriage'.

Are such attitudes still in existence within the police force? Of course, the answer is yes, not because the police are intrinsically woman hating, but because such attitudes exist within the wider society, of which police are a part, and from which recruits are drawn. There is much anecdotal evidence demonstrating an unhelpful and sometimes positively misogynist attitude by police officers towards women whom have been victims of violence at home. Comments such as 'If she were my wife I'd slap her', 'Go to bed and make it up', and 'There's no point in us coming out, you won't charge him, and you'll have him back when he's sober' have all been made by police officers in West Yorkshire and undoubtedly similar comments have been made all over the country. What effect do such attitudes have? Research such as that undertaken by Horley (1988) reveals that women often fail to report violent incidents because they believe that the police will not be sympathetic, helpful, or even come out to them in some cases. The idea has existed, certainly in the not too distant past if not now, that a violent marital incident is 'only a domestic', that will probably blow over, and therefore does not merit time spent getting statements from women who are never likely to proceed to court with their case. Little attention was paid to wondering why few cases ever reached the courts, or why some women repeatedly called the police but still remained in the marital home, waiting for the next time.

Why calling the police may not be the answer

As we have already seen, many women are themselves suffering from very low self-esteem as a result of being in an abusive relationship. This in itself can make them feel that they are partly responsible for what has happened, and therefore reluctant to involve the police, and to make public their own inadequacies as a wife. Many women genuinely care for their partners, and want to help them overcome their problems; they may regard calling the police as completely counter-productive when what their partner needs is tender, loving care and understanding. Lucy's story is typical of such a situation (see Figure 7.1).

Lucy's story

Lucy, a woman in her forties, had only recently married for the second time, after being a lone parent for ten years. Her first husband, a builder, had been a 'rough and ready' type – he had often spent the telephone money on alcohol, and would slap Lucy around if she complained, and he happened to be drunk at the time. Although he was quite a good father when he felt like being, as her children grew older, Lucy believed that they would benefit from more security in their lives, both emotionally and financially. Consequently, Lucy divorced her first husband, gained control of the finances and provided a happy stable environment for her children, for ten years. During that time, Lucy developed friendships rather than relationships, always putting her children first. Then she met Geoff. He was an educated man, an accountant, who had all the middle-class trappings that go with such occupations. More important than consumer items, however, was his gentle, thoughtful and considerate manner. Lucy was swept up by his charm and his sweet concern for her. Lucy had not mixed with many people from professional backgrounds, and she couldn't believe her luck. They were married within two months. On her return from the honeymoon, Lucy was slightly anxious – there had been an incident that had frightened her. Geoff had accused her of flirting with another holidaymaker and had flown into a rage. He had not hit her, but Lucy was scared that he would. She decided that Geoff had been badly scarred by a previous relationship, one in which he had been deserted in favour of someone else. She resolved to make him feel secure and loved, deciding that the way to do that was to work out what upset him and constantly reassure him. This turned out to be an impossible task, however. Geoff accused her of having an affair if she was longer at the shops than he thought necessary; he rang her every couple of hours to check on her whereabouts, and she became agitated if she had to speak to the teacher at school, in case she would be out when he next rang. As Geoff's behaviour became more and more irrational and unpredictable, Lucy's defence of him became more unrealistic. She believed that the more he was upset, even violent towards her, the more he was showing he trusted her with his innermost feelings and insecurities. She acknowledged that he needed help, but for quite a long time she believed that he needed her help. Consequently, when the violent attacks became more frequent and more dangerous (he tried to hit her with a hammer, and threw a brick through the window where she was sitting) there was absolutely no point in calling the police. Geoff was sick, not evil, he needed Lucy and she had to find a way to help him . Several months later, Lucy had to acknowledge that she could not give Geoff the support he needed. Lucy had to seek alternative accommodation in a different part of the town, so that Geoff would have no contact with her. She had to move her children to another school and eventually divorced Geoff. She later discovered that his last three relationships, including a twenty-year marriage, had all involved an horrendous amount of violence on his part.

Figure 7.1 Lucy's story

Obviously, the police would have been able to help Lucy in the midst of a dangerous incident, but for Lucy, the violence was a symptom of Geoff's insecurities. He was testing her, and she believed that if she had called the police, he would have regarded that as betraying him.

Social class may also play a factor in the decision to seek help – women from lower socio-economic groups may come from a culture in which the police are viewed suspiciously anyway, so they could not be considered part of a solution. Women from higher class backgrounds may be enveloped in an aura of disbelief. It can't be happening to them. It's only an isolated incident. Has some aspect of their own personality contributed to this? Whatever their thoughts, such women, especially young women, are frequently overcome with the enormity of such an event. Violence in middle-class relationships is rarely talked of, so many women prefer to end the relationship and move on, without ever formally acknowledging the violence by informing the police.

Can the police help?

If a woman is experiencing a violent attack by a partner, anyone can help. The woman can be helped out of the dangerous situation, the perpetrator can be restrained or removed – all necessary measures. If such measures are undertaken by the police, however, a message is being given that such behaviour is unacceptable to society as a whole, rather than an individual problem. How the police deal institutionally with various crimes is fundamentally important to how those activities are regarded by other members of society. For example, there may be some leniency shown by the police when they come into contact with young people in possession of cannabis, if the amount they have is obviously purely for personal use. The whole debate about legalisation or decriminalisation of the use of marijuana originates in the society as a whole, of which police are members, but the practices and attitudes that individual police officers may employ also fuels and influences general thinking. It is important to remember that police officers are also part of the society they police; as individuals they share many of the attitudes and prejudices that are generally held, and whilst they obviously have to work to strict guidelines, their underlying assumptions may sometimes be evident. For this reason, a welcome structural change in many forces has been the establishment of Domestic Violence Units.

Domestic Violence Units

These specialised units have been set up in many areas over the past eight years, or so. Their aim is to provide a service operated by police officers who are specifically trained in all of the issues relating to violence against women. Such training includes an understanding of the complex factors involved for many women, especially those with children. Officers are expected to listen to women, to work with them to achieve the most desirable outcome as chosen by the victim herself. For many women, this individual relationship with a supportive team of police officers can make all the difference in reviewing the possible options. Decisions about pressing charges, safety and preventative measures can all be considered in a reassuring setting. The police officers involved, and they can be both men and women, are committed to providing a non-judgmental and sympathetic social service, and for many, the establishment of such units has been a welcome development in both the acknowledgement and the eventual elimination of violence against women.

Criticisms of Domestic Violence Units

The very fact that a special unit has to be set up to deal with domestic violence has, for some, only emphasised the way that such crime is perceived as different from 'mainstream' violence. Critics argue that by addressing special attention to the abuse of women, it is seen as less important or relevant than violent crime dealt with through the usual procedures. Also, the existence of specially trained officers may release other police officers from having to think about the issues concerned with family violence. If it is seen as the responsibility of others, the basic, often negative, attitudes towards women may not be generally challenged, and domestic violence may continue to be marginalised and seen as less serious by the general population. Let us not forget that there have been many recent investigations into gross sexual harassment of women police officers by their male peers. If a misogynist culture exists among the police towards colleagues, it is difficult to see how an isolated special unit can change deep-rooted attitudes towards women in general.

The Women's Aid network

Women's Aid is a national organisation that provides temporary safe accommodation throughout Great Britain for women and their children who have experienced mental or physical harassment, or violence. It also offers support, help and advice to any woman, irrespective of whether or not she is resident in a refuge. Women's Aid also acts as a pressure group to educate and advise the wider society about the issue of domestic violence, acknowledging that the position of women in society is closely related and must also be addressed. The fundamental premise of Women's Aid is that it serves to encourage women to determine their own futures, whether this involves returning home or starting a new life. Whilst it recognises that women must decide for themselves a course of action, Women's Aid promotes the right for women to live in safety in their personal relationships.

The first officially recognised refuge was set up in 1969 by Erin Pizzey, in Chiswick. The publicity surrounding the provision of safe accommodation for women subjected to mental and physical abuse, resulted in the house being massively over-populated. Ms Pizzey declared that she would not send any woman away, and consequently, all the bedrooms, lounges and other available spaces were occupied. As the demand for such accommodation became obvious, women's groups all over the UK began to form under the banner of Women's Aid, to lobby local housing authorities to provide suitable buildings that could be used to house women and children.

The Women's Aid network operates an 'Open Door' policy, which means that any woman seeking refuge can be referred on to any other refuge in the country with available space, should she wish to move away, or if there is no space locally. For women and children who do seek refuge accommodation, no time limit is set on their stay, which can be as little as a few hours to however long it takes to secure permanent accommodation through the local authority housing department. Most refuges operate on self-help principles – residents are expected to cook, clean and generally run the accommodation. They are also encouraged to admit new residents, help them settle in and provide support to them, with the help of any paid or volunteer workers there may be. Such support may include accompanying women to solicitors' offices, to the courts, to housing departments, and so on. Women coming into a refuge are not regarded as clients who need to be helped – they are supported whilst they make their own decisions. Women are encouraged to play an active part in any decision making concerning the day-to-day running of the refuge. Through such participation, women are able to develop their confidence and self-esteem, which are likely to have been eroded through their experience of physical or mental abuse.

The emotional and educational needs of children are also acknowledged – most refuges have volunteer or paid workers whose main role is to work with the resident children. Such work involves helping mothers to care for and support their children in difficult circumstances, organising a whole range of activities to encourage the well-being and happiness of the children, and arranging placements in local schools for those who are old enough. The focus is on making a child's stay at a refuge as positive an experience as is possible. Occasionally, women enter a refuge whilst pregnant, and if they happen to still be living there after their baby has been born, they find an enormous wealth of support, concern and care shown to them by the other residents. The surroundings may need a lick of paint, the baby clothes may all be second hand, but the emotional bonds between the women are immeasurable.

Other help offered by Women's Aid

So far we have concentrated on the support offered to women and their children who seek refuge accommodation, but Women's Aid does, in fact, offer its services throughout the country to women who do not want or need to seek alternative living arrangements as well. Any woman can seek advice, support, reassurance or simply a break from isolation by telephoning either the local or national network. Workers at refuges have helped many, many women whom they never meet, and outreach centres are also available in some towns, where women can drop in whenever they want to. Many local groups also offer aftercare assistance for women who have come through the refuge system – continuing support both from the refuge workers and, perhaps more significantly, from other women who have also had similar experiences.

Negative aspects of Women's Aid and refuge provision? – thinking the unthinkable?

One of the advantages of there being an umbrella organisation to which most refuges are affiliated, is that there are national guidelines to which all local branches adhere; these include principles such as always accepting as true what women say about their experiences, and being aware that a refuge must not continue to make a women feel inadequate, by taking over her life and making the 'right' decision as viewed by others.

For many women in a violent relationship, having nowhere to go has been a contributory factor in their remaining in such a situation. Staying with family or friends is often a temporary solution, and can also cause more anxiety if women are worried about putting others at risk. It is not uncommon for violent men to seek out their partners, and as they may be in a charged emotional state, others may feel threatened or even experience violence towards themselves or their property. The mere knowledge of the existence of refuges may constrain a violent man's behaviour, if he realises that his partner could leave him, even taking their children, and that there need be no physical or emotional dependence on him at all, thereby reducing his power.

Identifying the need for refuge provision, and implementing the establishment of such accommodation, has therefore had a major impact on the lives of thousands of women. However, the 'supply' of refuges has been far outstripped by the 'demand' for places within them – a measure of their success but also a factor that generates its own set of problems. Refuges are often poorly funded, situated in sub-standard housing, and, most significantly, overcrowded, which can lead to stress, depression and even result in a women returning to a violent relationship.

Of course, some women will always want to return to their partners, to try again, and a refuge can give a woman the time to sort out her own emotional needs. However, when it is the structural problems within a refuge that influence a woman's decision, it is unacceptable. The lack of governmental commitment to refuge provision can be evidenced by the fact that to date there are only about 200 refuges throughout the United Kingdom, despite the fact that the Government Select Committee on Violence and Marriage recommended one family place per 10,000 of the population (Women's Aid Federation, 1992) which should result in over 5000 refuges. This could be interpreted as a clear indication of the ideology of patriarchy at the root of the Establishment. Lip-service acceptance of the need for alternative accommodation may suggest an underlying belief in the importance of maintaining the family unit, even when members of that unit are at risk.

Ideological influence from external sources is at best unhelpful; ideological positions within the movement itself can be completely destructive. In an effort perhaps, to establish themselves as professional agencies, and thereby worthy of funding, some refuges may have developed their role as advisers to a greater extent, thereby rendering the women coming into refuges as clients in need of a service. Whilst this may seem normal, even a good thing perhaps, it can subtly reinforce the low self-esteem of women who have already lost much of their confidence in their abilities. Women may turn to staff members to sort out their benefit forms, or their housing applications and this can detract from the enabling situation of taking control of their own lives, albeit with support from others. Becoming seen as a professional agency may have done wonders for the credibility of Women's Aid as a movement, and has undoubtedly raised the issue of violence against women, but have the needs of women fleeing violence been served? Consider the links between refuges and their funding bodies: refuges are a financial asset to whoever owns them, and the structure of the building must therefore be maintained. Due to the fluctuating nature of the body of residents, this may result in staff members either taking control of tasks such as decorating (thereby establishing the hierarchy within the refuge) or enforcing rules and rotas, whereby residents are expected to carry out certain duties. Clearly, rules about hygiene and general living arrangements are vital in a multiple occupancy household, but what about rules about house keys or going out at night time? What about the children in a refuge – should there be rules about bed times, and so on ? In whose interest are rules made – those of the residents or of the institution itself?

Power structures

Every institution, from the most private (family) to the most public (a multi-national corporation) is prey to the forces of institutionalisation, whereby structures and procedures appear to take on a life of their own, and are carried out in particular ways, because they have always been done like that. Perhaps due to the awareness of such a tendency, most refuges will endorse democratic procedures; one example being regular meetings between residents and staff, at which the former can raise issues they are concerned about. However, such visible exchanges of views are often dominated by what Lukes (1974) calls the 'third dimension of power', the invisible influence of the institution which actually leads to the acceptance of any underlying ideology without question. This may lead women to believe that there is a 'desired outcome' of their situation, and that any choice other than leaving their violent partner would be seen as less acceptable. Residents may also be aware of the 'second dimension' of power, where others, usually staff members, control the agenda, i.e., decide what issues to genuinely discuss. Despite claims from workers in the refuge movement, there is an undeniable power imbalance between themselves and the women they serve, which it may be possible to address, but only if it is first recognised. Inequalities exist within all groups, but they can be compounded by the denial of their existence. Whilst gender is seen to be a unifying factor within Women's Aid, the significance of class and ethnicity are often overlooked. As we have already noted, many women from lower socio-economic groups come into a refuge, often because of the lack of financial resources to seek alternative solutions. Such women may have already been disadvantaged by their class position. Inequalities within the education system may have channelled them into low-paid jobs with little status and little opportunity to develop an idea of their self-worth. Practices that exist within the refuge movement can further undermine their ability to help themselves. Solicitors, teachers, doctors and housing officials all tend to demonstrate middle-class values, often through the use of language and their interaction. If women in refuges are accompanied by the acceptable face of the Women's Movement (the salaried employee), this can reinforce the class differential and thereby underpin the structural weakness inherent in the social and economic position of many working-class women. It is obviously difficult to balance the desire to help, with the need to let others help themselves.

The experiences of black women have also been a cause for concern within Women's Aid and other refuge providers. Racial discrimination has been a factor, as suggested by Mama (1989), both in terms of the assistance offered to black women and also racism (overt as well as 'unintended'). To address this, some refuges have been set up by black women for black women so that these women do not experience the 'triple jeopardy' of being a woman, being poor and being black.

These criticisms of the refuge movement certainly do not detract from its position at the forefront of the fight for women to live in a safe environment, but they do focus attention on the fact that no organisation should be complacent, however well meaning it aims to be.

Treatment for the abusers and the abused

Women and therapy

We have seen that violence against women is part of a wider pattern of social interaction, which locates men in a much more powerful position than women. If we acknowledge this, can any treatment or therapy aimed at individuals be of any use? It depends, perhaps, on both the purpose of the therapy, and the rationale behind it. If, for example, therapy is used to help women who have experienced violence to move on from a bad situation, to recreate themselves as capable, independent women, then it can obviously be of great benefit. If women become aware of the patriarchal forces that often shape their identity and their interactions, then they can be more in control of both.

Couples and therapy

Couples who voluntarily agree to put themselves forward for therapy may also gain a clearer understanding of their own relationship and the roles they play within it. Care must be taken, however, to ensure that joint therapy is not equated with joint responsibility for the violence. Goldner (1991), in her work with such couples, insists that the man admit responsibility for his violence and pledges unconditionally to stop using violence. Sessions include examining the upbringing of each person, and the extent to which gender roles are perceived as relevant. For many women, Goldner notes that the notion of nurturing and caring for their partners is frequently uppermost in their minds; they feel they must continue to help their partners even when they have been violent towards them. Goldner believes part of her work with couples is to encourage the women to question and perhaps reassess their gender roles, and to make it clear that violence will not be tolerated under any circumstances. Exploring their beliefs and reactions in this way can lead to new ways of relating to each other, or can result in the permanent separation of the couple. Both consequences are valid if they lead to a challenging of the assumptions behind violent behaviour and an awareness that it is possible to change the way individuals respond in particular situations.

Men and therapy

It is less common for men who use violence against their partners to seek help or treatment. This may be for a number of reasons: they may be unable to articulate their feelings about emotional issues, due to their socialisation; they may be worried what others will think about them if they admit such behaviour; or they may quite simply refuse to accept responsibility for what has happened, by blaming either their partners or inanimate causes, such as alcohol or stress. A basic tenet of therapy or re-education programmes is that perpetrators of violence do acknowledge that they have committed the violent acts and that they, and only they, were responsible. Exploration of their ideas about masculinity and how it is demonstrated through 'macho' behaviour are common issues discussed in such sessions, as are alternative means of expressing maleness in ways that do not inflict harm on others. These ideas are developed from the psycho-analytical approach, whereby the root cause of behaviour is sought in an attempt to understand why it occurs. Another approach, which comes perhaps from the behavioural school, is that of anger management, in which men using violence are considered to have been inadequately socialised and therefore need to learn techniques for controlling their anger. They are also taught to become aware of trigger factors that may spark off violent incidents, and learn how to use particular strategies to deflect or dissipate such negative feelings.

Adam Jukes (1993), who has worked extensively with male abusers, however, claims that whilst trust is an important issue in the treatment of such men:

> it is not possible to trust a batterer ... experience of trusting men has taught me a painful lesson: not that batterers cannot be trusted at all, but that it is impossible to know which can be trusted and when. (1993:307)

Many men who attended re-education programmes, and were expressing positive ideas about their behaviour, were in fact still subjecting their partners to violent outbursts. Jukes maintains that the involvement of the police, the use of the law and a system of therapy and re-education programmes should all be combined to provide the most effective means for preventing violence against women.

The force of the law gives, as we have said, a clear public statement about the unacceptability of domestic violence. If all men who were violent to their partners were summarily charged with assault, and hence experienced the public disapproval of their behaviour, which many of them fear, they may be thus encouraged to seek psychological help to understand and ultimately prevent their behaviour. Individual remedies for violent behaviour need to be set in the wider context of the society that currently colludes with, perhaps even causes the behaviour of the family criminal.

In each chapter of this book the enormous complexity of both domestic violence and the systems in place to deal with that violence has been illustrated. There are no easy answers, nor simple quick-fix solutions. To suggest a woman leaves her family home and moves into a refuge is a major decision, with long-lasting consequences.

This chapter has examined some of the ways in which some women can be helped as they live in violent and abusive relationships. Throughout the book, it has become clear that domestic violence is a complex issue. There are no universal solutions and there is no universal experience or response to violence. All midwives should be aware of what is available and should know the advantages and disadvantages of various solutions and actions. In the final chapter, we will draw some conclusions.

Chapter 8

Summary and conclusions

*Domestic violence is not a comfortable topic.
Patients do not find it easy to raise. Staff may
be anxious about their ability to respond. Too
often the problem remains undisclosed; no
appropriate response is offered; no effective
intervention is made.*

(Department of Health, Domestic Violence website)

The main issues

In this chapter we will seek to draw out the main issues and concerns that we have raised in the book. In addition, we will set the issue of domestic violence in its social policy context. Of particular importance are the actions being undertaken by the Home Office and the Department of Health. The policies of the 1997 Labour Government have been different to those of previous administrations; at least domestic violence is now being considered and an attempt is being made to ensure that different departments of government are working together.

Domestic violence is a crime. Associating the crime with its location, in this case, the home, risks sanitising both the criminal and the action. Violence is a crime, regardless of when or where or how it is committed. The Department of Health website (http://doh.gov.uk/domviol.htm), states that domestic violence refers to the physical, sexual or emotional abuse inflicted on a spouse or partner by the other. They usually live together but this need not be the case. The vast majority of victims are women and the perpetrators men; but men may be victims and domestic violence can also occur where both partners are of the same sex. The Department of Health urges staff to be alert to the problem, understand the legal context and know how to respond.

Domestic violence is a major public health issue in the United Kingdom and all over the world. As such it must be everyone's business and, in particular, the business of health professionals. It is clearly our problem, not the problem of some other agency or authority. Midwives have a key role in the health of women and their children and, as such, they must play a pivotal role in society's response to this abuse of women.

It is only when midwives openly acknowledge that all women and children are potential victims that we can begin to change the nature of society and its attitudes.

In this book we have considered the nature of domestic violence and sought to separate the physical effects from the emotional and psychological effects. We have debated the incidence of domestic violence and justified our stance to focus mainly on the needs of women rather than men. We have noted that battered women come from all backgrounds and lifestyles, but all have low self-esteem, feel inadequate, believe that they are responsible for the violence and generally feel that no one could help them except themselves.

Much of this book has focused on the shape and very nature of the society in which we live and work. We have tried to help the reader examine and ask questions about sex and gender. We have considered the root source of aggression and the biological explanations that are used as excuses for male violence. We have considered the open acceptability of violence, the blind eye we turn when a child is physically hit in a busy shopping centre, or when a child is threatened with violence by an older more powerful controlling adult who exerts his or her power physically in an attempt to socialise a child into acceptable behaviour.

What is clear is that domestic violence is a complex problem and there are no quick fix solutions. For midwives, there is an overwhelming need to consider the complexities of violence in close couple relationships and to avoid the trap of telling a woman what she must do, reinforced by a firmly voiced statement about what you as a midwife would do in that situation. It is far more difficult to listen, support, understand and do nothing than it is to direct, control and add insult to injury by belittling, criticising and be despairing of a woman who has chosen to share her experiences.

Diane's story (see Figure 8.1) is a long one, but it successfully illustrates some of the complexities of a relationship and life history dominated by domestic violence. Based on an interview with Diane, this story clarifies many of the concepts that this book addresses. It charts the development of domestic violence, describes the trigger factors, explores the complexities of the decision to leave an abusive relationship and describes the consequences of violence. It examines the midwife's response or lack of response to her experience of violence. It is a sobering and true story.

Diane's story

Diane is 35 years old and pregnant with her fifth child. She was married at 18; her eldest son is 17. The violence began some twenty years ago. She met Michael when she was 14, at a time when she was confused and upset by the discovery that the person she had called her mother all her life was in fact her grandmother and her older sister was really her mother. Michael offered stability and comfort. The relationship was intense and passionate. In fact, even at that early stage Michael said that if ever Diane left him, he would kill her. He was controlling and aggressive. Diane believes she saw him as a father figure but also as a man who wanted to own and possess her. He resented her relationships with other members of her family, always criticising them for her childhood.

Diane said:

I didn't realise it, but he was stopping me from having my freedom right from the start. I was not allowed to see my friends. It was done in such a way that I was made to feel that I was abusing him or letting him down by giving them time. I was confused. I could not understand why he was so possessive. I found myself making excuses to my family.

The violence was mostly verbal to start with – endless rows, over minor things. He kept it up for days at a time. It usually started because I was a long time at the shops. He would accuse me of flirting. He never hit me then but he would grab me around my throat to frighten me. He said it was to shut me up.

Diane explained that if ever she hinted that the relationship had gone sour or that she wanted to leave he would say that he loved her and could not go on without her. He would say that he would die if she left. Diane never admitted to herself that she was already too frightened to leave.

As the years went by, Diane had more children and as a family they were more deeply in debt. Unemployment hit the family and Diane started to steal to feed the children.

Michael was really impressed with Diane's success in stealing. He would lavish praise on her and boast to his friends of her achievements. Eventually she was caught and put on probation. The family were even more in debt. Diane was pregnant and the physical violence began. Diane said:

When I was first pregnant he became physically violent and he really hurt me badly. I had black eyes regularly. He would punch me in the stomach and in the heat of the argument he would try to strangle me.

> *After the violence, he was full of remorse. He would cry and say: 'How can I have done this to you?' He would never give me flowers or anything but he made me feel that he loved me so much. Then he would make out it was my fault. He would say: 'If you hadn't said that or if you hadn't done that ...'.*

Diane would try to explain that her actions were normal, but in the end she would apologise just to calm things down. She explained that she always believed that she could change the situation. She spent her life believing that she could change Michael, but eventually she said:

> *I always thought that I could change things, I never could. You can only change yourself not someone else.*

Later in the interview Diane went on to explain that the violence in pregnancy really did frighten her. It was as if she could bear injuries to herself but not to her unborn child. Injuries to her breasts and abdomen were common but all her children were born healthy.

Diane said:

> *When I had the bruises and the black eyes, I was not allowed to go to the clinic. He stopped me until they had healed. If the midwife came to the house, I was not allowed to answer the door. When I went to the clinic I wore lots of make up. I never wanted the midwives to know about violence, even when my back was aching because of a punch more than the pregnancy. The scans were okay; the monitoring of the heart beat was fine, so no one took any notice of the bruises. No one ever asked me if I was okay, or if I was being abused. I didn't expect them to, and I probably would not have told them anyway.*

Asked about the pattern of violence, Diane said:

> *There is a pattern, a row, I could always sense it. I would say the wrong thing or I would do something wrong. It was often when he had a hangover, but not always. I would avoid him then. He was tense, irritable, then the explosion would come. He would keep me up all night long. It didn't matter to him – he could sleep all day, but I had the kids to see to.*

I was very, very stressed, worn out in fact. I was crying out for help, desperate. I didn't know where to turn. The tension got worse and worse. Then he would hit me, hit me, kick me. Anything. Then it would be over.

Then followed the remorse. I was always kept a prisoner. Then, I was not even allowed to go to the shops. He was worried I would run away. If we needed anything, he would send the kids. This would go on until he was sure I would not run away. I did run away. I went to my sister and to my mother. I have left him lots of times. He wrote me long love letters, full of remorse – 'Give me another chance', 'I'll never do it again'. I always felt that I owed him another chance, so I went back. We would go through this honeymoon period. We pretended we were in love. He would be a good husband and father. He would improve, but slowly the same old pattern returned.

There was always emotional blackmail. He would use the children, saying how unhappy they would be without him. He did not provide for them, but he did love them. He would use the children to get us back together, demanding that they put pressure on me. It always worked and when I felt guilty I would come back. The refuges were awful and the kids are important.

Diane explained how often she had left him and stayed in hostels or with her family:

At least twenty times, I have been close to a nervous breakdown, I have stayed in at least twenty hostels.

She described her injuries:

I have had a dislocated shoulder. He broke my finger. He hit me on the head with the heel of his shoe. I have never been to hospital. It has never been that serious – just bruising, black eyes, strangling marks around my neck, nothing too serious. He used to try not to mark my face. It would be obvious to other people. It was my breasts, my back, just his fists, no weapons except the heel of his shoe; he used to throw chairs and tables but no weapons.

One particular time stands out in my mind. I was curled up in the corner and he got my son to pour a cup of blackcurrant juice over me. He was three years old. I was curled up in the corner, then he told him to wee on me. I was so humiliated; that is something I have never forgiven. My son is lost now; he will never respect women.

I stayed for the children really; now I know how much it damages the children. I didn't then. As I got stronger, I started to read books about violent men. Men are little babies in a way, insecure, boys who are not grown up. I worked hard to make it right, but being abused drains your energy; it used up all my resources.

The decision to leave him for good has taken a long time, I always knew that I could not spend the rest of my life with him, but it was never the right time. It was always the children; I was always pregnant, but now it is different. I have started divorce proceedings, but he still comes every week for his dinner, to see the children. He is still manipulating me from his flat. He still asks the children where I am going, who am I seeing. He rings; he writes begging letters; he threatens to kill himself, but I have got to get on with my life. Its always when I say I am going to leave that he threatens to kill me, this is the time when I am most afraid.

I hope this new baby is a boy, I can teach him how to respect women; it's too late for the others. I want to bring this one up on my own. When I have finished I am going to go to college. I want a fresh start, a new life without a man.

Diane is still living apart from Michael and is determined to start a new life alone. The path ahead is neither clear nor easy, but she is determined it will be a different life from the one she has had in the past.

Figure 8.1 Diane's story

It would be easy to fall into the trap of believing that Diane's problems were associated with her social class, her poverty, her anti-social behaviour (the stealing of food for her children) and alcohol abuse, but that would be wrong. Violence is common across all social classes, all ethnic groups, all age groups and not confined to man/woman relationships. Women who are abused are not victims but, as Diane's story illustrates, the incredible survivors of an impossible situation. We fail to honour the position of women in such relationships if we do not recognise the complexities and conflicting demands made on women. This story is important in that it reminds us that women we meet as midwives may have been in an abusive situation for many years and have been subjected to physical, sexual and emotional abuse. It also reminds us that women are not always free agents, free to walk away from abusive relationships. Diane's story illustrates how she was trapped financially and how she tried many different ways of stopping the violence. Finally, it illustrates how the period of greatest danger can be around the time a woman decides to leave.

It is increasingly clear that midwives have a key role to play in supporting women who are in abusive relationships. The midwife has a unique opportunity to be non-judgmental, supportive, kind and understanding. Building on the unique relationship of trust that she has established with a woman during her childbearing experience, she can support the woman in whatever decision she makes, recognising the multiplicity of factors involved and complexity of that process. It is so easy to take control and tell a woman to leave the relationship. It is so difficult to stand alongside as an equal and respect her right to make a decision that on the surface seems unreasonable and even stupid. Midwives must also consider that when a woman discloses domestic violence it may have taken her many years to find the courage to discuss it. It may also be that the midwife is one of many 'professionals' who have failed to respond adequately to her story. Midwives should always remember that many women trust them implicitly. Abused women are likely to remember what the midwife says and how she says it. They are also likely to be acutely sensitive to any advice that the midwife offers.

The Government response to domestic violence

When the Labour Government was elected in May 1997 it was expected that issues of injustice would be tackled in a more enthusiastic manner than during the previous Tory administration. Domestic violence suffers from being a woman's issue and, as we have seen in previous chapters, women's issues take second place to those of men. The Government has, in fact, made domestic violence a priority and has created a minister for women, currently Margaret Jay. In June 1999 Jack Straw, the Home Secretary, in response to the setting up of a new magistrates court dealing solely with domestic violence, said:

> *Like racial harassment, domestic violence is one of those rare fields where we want to see an increase in recorded crime. We have left the dark ages when people were told to stop bothering the police over 'mere domestics', but it isn't acceptable that it takes on average 35 alleged assaults before a case comes to court.*
> (*The Guardian*, 3 June, 1999).

The Home Office has devised a strategy called 'Living without Fear'. This is seen as an integrated approach to tackling violence against women. The strategy can be criticised in that it seeks to co-ordinate responses and disseminate examples of good practice without any additional funding and without tackling the inequalities in our society that we have already described. The new strategy is available on a website (http://www.cabinet-office.gov.uk/women's-unit/1999/fear/03.htm). Theoretically, this makes the strategy more open and more available to those who are trying to help. Chapter one of the strategy, 'Setting the scene', sets out the Government's commitment to make domestic violence a public issue and not one that is swept under the carpet. The strategy is built on three pillars, protection and provision, justice and prevention and recognises the scale of the problem. The Government promises women that they will follow up with a publicity campaign, the new leaflet *Breaking the Chain*, raise awareness in schools and the wider community, expand the Victim Support Witness Service and offer vulnerable or intimidated witnesses better protection in the courts. The proof of the pudding will be in the eating, but at last Government does seem to be taking domestic violence seriously.

The new NHS – modern and dependable

In December 1997 the Government issued a White paper, *The New NHS*. It set out the Government's intention to modernise the NHS. The first task was to abolish the internal market and replace that bureaucracy with another. This time a more integrated system would build on partnerships between health, social care and voluntary agencies. There is to be greater accountability, more partnerships, a reduction in bureaucracy and a gradual rebuilding of public confidence in the NHS. In the first stages, local health authorities were required to design locally based health improvement programmes, Health Action Zones were to be established, primary care groups and teams were to be set up and establishing clinical governance became a priority for Trusts. The Public Health Green Paper, *Our Healthier Nation*, was published in 1998. Here it was acknowledged that people's health was affected by their circumstances. The Social Exclusion Unit was set up to tackle such issues as poverty and teenage pregnancy. The Labour Government clearly has a public health agenda and tackling domestic violence is part of that agenda.

Making a difference

In the autumn of 1999 the Department of Health launched the strategy for nursing and midwifery. The document was subtitled *Strengthening the nursing, midwifery and health visiting contribution to health and healthcare*. The strategy recognised the changing context of care and the need for nurses and midwives to respond to a policy that sought to modernise the NHS. Probably for the first time, public health rather than illness was exercising the minds of politicians. The needs of local communities and local strategies to address local needs have become the order of the day. Apart from chapters that set out reforms to recruitment, education, the new consultant nurse and midwife, and professional regulation, Chapter 10, called *Working in new ways*, describes the proposals to expand the role of midwives. The chapter recognises midwives' skills and the therapeutic relationship they already can establish with women during pregnancy. The Government wants to expand the role of the midwife and make better use of her skills in all aspects of women's health. Midwives must play a key role in tackling inequalities in health and targeting vulnerable groups. Postnatal depression, breast feeding, and lifestyle advice are all areas in which midwives can make a difference. Postnatal examination, family planning, psychological and social problems all become part of the midwife's role. Tackling domestic violence is clearly a major new area for midwifery intervention. This book has made the case for midwives to get involved and provided them with some of the skills and knowledge they need. The reward for midwives will be the establishment of midwifery consultant posts, where a salary of £40,000 is promised.

Back at the Trust

It is important that every NHS Trust with maternity services has a clear policy for training midwives to ask direct questions about domestic violence and a clear policy as to the action a midwife should take when domestic violence is disclosed. Midwives need training to help them support the one in four women who are abused in pregnancy. Multi-professional education, working in partnership with managers, social workers and the professions allied to medicine will be beneficial. They need to be supported themselves by managers and supervisors of midwives. Midwives need to feel safe and be sure that there are Trust policies in place that will keep them safe. First, midwives need to examine their own attitudes to domestic violence and consider if deep down they still believe that abuse is the woman's fault, or if her decision to stay in an abusive relationship means the midwife should wash her hands of the case.

Every maternity unit should arrange for information on domestic violence to be printed on the maternity records that are held by the woman. Local and national telephone numbers and help lines should be printed on notes and on posters in public areas and posted in ladies toilets and examination rooms.

Only when it is recognised that domestic violence is everyone's business, and that its roots lie in the sexist nature of our patriarchal society will we begin to recognise and deal with this heinous crime.

CHESTER COLLEGE LIBRARY

Women's Aid
PO Box 391, Bristol BS99 7WS
0117 944 4411.

Women's Aid National Domestic Violence Helpline
0345 023 468.

Refuges 24-hour national Crisis Line
0990 995 443.

Victim Support Line
0845 30 30 900.

Black Association of Women Step Out Ltd (BAWSO)
Aims to offer a holistic service to all visible ethnic minority women and children in Wales
01222 343154.

Beverley Lewis House
PO Box 7312, London, E15 4TS
A refuge which provides safe accommodation for women with learning disabilities
020 8522 0675.

Southall Black Sisters
Provides a comprehensive and holistic service to Asian and African-Caribbean women
020 8571 9595.

Newham Asian Women's Project
020 8472 0528.

The Survivors Directory
Lists support and counselling services for survivors of sexual abuse
0161 277 7000.

Miles Beale
020 7 270 6454;
fax 020 7270 6253.
Funding from the Invest to Save Budget to develop projects that bring together public bodies to deliver innovative services to support women.

References

Abbey B, Berenson M D, San Miguel V V, Wilkinson G S (1992), 'Prevalence of Physical And Sexual Assault In Pregnant Adolescents', *Journal of Adolescent Health*, 13, pp 466-469.

Abbott P and Wallace C (1997), *An Introduction to Sociology (Feminist Perspectives)*, London, Routledge.

Acheson D (1998), *Independent Inquiry Into Inequalities in Health Report*, Chairman Sir Donald Acheson, London, The Stationery Office.

Amaro H, Fried L E, Cabral H, Zurcherman B (1990), 'Violence during pregnancy and substance abuse', *American Journal of Public Health*, 80, pp 575-579.

Andrews B and Brown G W (1988), 'Marital Violence in the community: A Biographical Approach', *British Journal of Psychiatry*, 153, pp 305-312.

Anthias F and Yuval Davis N (1993), *Racialised Boundaries*, London, Routledge.

Archer J and Lloyd B (1989), *Sex and Gender*, Harmondsworth, Penguin.

Backett K C (1980), 'Images of Parenthood' in M Anderson (ed), *Sociology of the Family*, Harmondsworth, Penguin.

Bakowski M, Murch M and Walker V (1983), *Marital Violence: The Community Response*, London, Tavistock Publications.

Barker M (1981), *New Racism*, London, Junction Books.

Berenson A B, Wiemann C M, Wilkinson G S, Jones W A and Anderson G D (1994), 'Perinatal Morbidity Associated With Violence Experienced by Pregnant Women', *American Journal of Obstetrics and Gynecology*, 170, pp 1760-1769.

Berne E (1968), *Games People Play*, Harmondsworth, Penguin.

Bewley C A and Gibbs A (1991), 'Violence in Pregnancy', *Midwifery*, 7, pp 107-112.

Bewley C A and Gibbs A (1997), 'The Role of the Midwife' in S Bewley, J Friend, G Mezey (eds) (1997), *Violence against Women*, London, Royal College of Obstetricians and Gynaecologists.

Bewley C A and Gibbs A (2000), 'Domestic Violence and Pregnancy' in Jo Alexander, Carolyn Roth and Valerie Levy (eds), *Midwifery Practice Core Topics 3*, Basingstoke, Macmillan.

Bewley S, Friend J, Mezey G (eds) (1997), *Violence against Women*, London, Royal College of Obstetricians and Gynaecologists.

Binney V, Harkell G and Nixon J (1981), *Leaving Violent Men: a Study of Refuges and Housing for Battered Women*, Leeds, Women's Aid Federation.

Birke L (1992), 'In Pursuit of Difference' in G Kirkup and L Smith-Keller (eds), *Inventing Women*, Cambridge, Polity Press.

'Blackstone's Commentary on the Laws of England (1765)', cited in Bourlet A (1990), *Police Intervention in Marital Violence*, Milton Keynes, Open University Press.

Bohn D (1990), 'Domestic Violence and Pregnancy Implications for Practice', *Journal of Nurse Midwifery*, 35, No. 2, pp 86-88.

Bott E (1971), *Family and Social Networks*, Second Edition, London, Tavistock.

Bourlet A (1990), *Police Intervention in Marital Violence*, Milton Keynes, Open University Press.

Bowker L H (1983), *Beating Wife Beating*, Lexington, Lexington Books.

Boyd J and Klingbeil K (1993) cited in S Schornstein (1997), *Domestic Violence and Healthcare: What Every Professional Needs To Know*, New York, Sage Publications.

Bradshaw M (1987), 'Attitudinal Abuse Towards Pregnant Women', *Holistic Nursing Practice*, 1, No. 2, pp 1-12.

Brewer E C (1978), *The Dictionary of Phrase and Fable*, New York, Avenal Books.

BMA (British Medical Association) (1998), *Domestic Violence*, London, BMA.

Britten N and Heath A (1983), 'Women, Men and Social Class' in E Garmarnikow, D Morgan, J Purvis and D Taylorson, *Gender, Class and Work*, London, Heinemann.

Brown J (1996), 'The Process of Change For Abused Women, Stages of Change' in P A Paluzzi and L Slattery, *No Woman Deserves To Hurt. Domestic Violence Education For Women's Health Care Providers*, USA, American College of Nurse-Midwives.

Browne K (1993), *An Introduction to Sociology*, Cambridge, Polity Press.

Bullock L F and McFarlane J (1989), 'The Birth Weight/Battering Connection', *American Journal of Nursing*, No. 89, pp 1153-1155.

Butterworth T and Faugier J (1996), *Clinical Supervision and Mentorship in Nursing*, London, Chapman & Hall.

Campbell J C, Oliver C, Bullock L (1993), 'Why Battering During Pregnancy?', *Clinical Issues in Women's Health Nursing 4*, pp 343-349.

Campbell J, Millar P and Cardwell M M (1994), 'Relationship Status of Battered Women Over Time', *Journal of Family Violence*, 9, pp 99-111.

Campbell R and Macfarlane A (1994), *Where To Be Born? The Debate and the Evidence*, Oxford, National Perinatal Epidemiology Unit.

Chagnon B (1968) in J Pahl (ed) (1985) *Private Violence and Public Policy: The Needs of Battered Women and the Responses of the Public Services*, London, Routledge and Kegan Paul.

Chaney J (1981), *Social Networks and Job Information: The Situation of Women Who Return to Work*, Report presented to the Equal Opportunities Commission.

Chodorow N (1978), *The Reproduction of Mothering*, Berkeley, University of California Press.

Churcher J (1997) in J Okely (1983), *The Traveller-Gypsies*, Cambridge, Cambridge University Press.

Cochrane L (1997), 'Mothers To Be Face Increased Risk of Violence', *Scotsman*, 3, May 2.

Colgan K (1995), *You Have to Scream With Your Mouth Shut*, Dublin, Marino Books.

Connors KA, Heisner L and Trickett P (1992), 'CAPINEX: Abstract descriptors', *Journal of Family Violence*, No. 4, pp 321-334.

Covington D L, Dalton V K, Diehl S J, *et al.* (1997), 'Improving Detection of Violence Among Pregnant Adolescents', *Journal of Adolescent Health*, 21, No. 1, July, pp 18-24.

Criminal Statistics for England and Wales 1996, http://www.homeoffice.gov.uk/cpd/cpsu/domviol98.htm

Curry M A, Doyle B A, Gilhooley J (1998), 'Abuse Among Pregnant Adolescents. Differences by Developmental Age', *MCN*, 23, No. 3 May/June 1998, pp 144-150.

Davidson A (1998), *Taking Control of Our Life in Stages*, Conference Paper, 'Domestic Violence - A Fresh Approach' RCOG, 25 July .

Davies C (1995), *Gender and the Professional Predicament in Nursing*, Buckingham, Open University Press.

De Beauvoir S (1952/1974), *The Second Sex*, Harmondsworth, Penguin.

Delphy C (1984), *Close to Home: A Materialist Analysis of Women's Oppression*, London, Hutchinson.

DoH (Department of Health) (1993), *Changing Childbirth; Part 1 The Report of the Expert Advisory Group*, London, HMSO.

Department of Health, Welsh Office, Scottish Office DoH, DoH and SS Northern Ireland, *Why Mothers Die: Report on Confidential Enquiries into Maternal Deaths in the United Kingdom 1994-1996*, London, The Stationery Office.

Department of Health (1997), http://www.doh.gov.uk/domviol.htm

Dex S (1985), *The Sexual Division of Work*, Brighton, Wheatsheaf.

Dimond B (1994), *The Legal Aspects of Midwifery*, Cheshire, England, Books for Midwives Press.

Dinnerstein D (1987), *The Rocking of the Cradle and the Ruling of the World*, London, The Women's Press.

Dobash E R and Dobash R P (1979), *Violence Against Wives*, Shepton Mallett, Open Books.

Dobash E R and Dobash R P (1991), *Women, Violence and Social Change*, London, Routledge.

Dominy N and Radford L (1996), *Domestic Violence in Surrey: Towards an Effective Inter-Agency Response*, Surrey Social Services, Roehampton Institute.

Dublin Women's Aid (1993), 'How Not To Be An Abused/Battered Woman', in K Colgan (1995), *You Have to Scream With Your Mouth Shut*, Dublin, Marino Books.

Durrani T (1996), *My Feudal Lord*, London, Corgi Books.

Edgell S (1980), *Middle Class Couples*, London, Allen and Unwin.

Edwards S (1997), 'The Law and Domestic

Violence' in S Bewley, J Friend, G Mezey (eds), *Violence Against Women*, London, RCOG Press.

Ehlers C L, Rickler K C, and Hovey J E (1980), 'A Possible Relationship Between Plasma Testosterone and Aggressive Behaviour in a Female Outpatient Population' in M Giris and L G Kiloh (eds), *Limbic Epilepsy and the Dyscontrol Syndrome*, New York, Elsevier.

Fawcett B, Featherstone B, Hearn J, Toft C (eds) (1996), *Violence and Gender Relations* Wiltshire, Cromwell Press.

Freud S (1920/1975), *Beyond the Pleasure Principle*, 1975 Edition, New York, Norton.

Garmarnikow E (1983), *Gender, Class and Work*, London, Heinemann.

Gayford J J (1978) 'Battered Wives', in J P Martin (ed), *Violence and the Family*, New York, John Wiley and Sons.

Gazmararian J, Lazorick S, Sptiz A, Ballard T, Saltzman L and Marks J (1996), 'Prevalence of Violence Against Pregnant Women', *Journal of American Medical Association*, 275, pp 1915-1919.

Gazmararian J, Lazorick S, Sptiz A, Ballard T, Saltzman L and Marks J (1996), 'Prevalence of Violence Against Pregnant Women', *Journal of the American Medical Association*, 275, pp 1915-1919.

Gelles R J (1974), *The Violent Home*, Beverly Hills, CA, Sage Publications.

Gelles R J (1987), *Family Violence*, 2nd edition, Newbury Park, CA, Sage Publications.

Gielen A C , O'Campo P J, Faden R R, Kass N E, Xue X (1994), 'Interpersonal conflict and physical violence during the childbearing year', *Social Science and Medicine*, 39, pp 781-787.

Goldner V (1991), 'Sex, Power and Gender: A Feminist Systematic Analysis of the Politics of Passion', *Journal of Feminist Family Therapy*, 3, pp 63-83.

Goldthorpe J H (1980), *Social Mobility and Class Structure in Modern Britain*, Oxford, Clarendon Press.

Grabrucker M (1988), *There's a Good Girl: Gender Stereotyping in the First Three Years of Life*, London, The Women's Press.

Gross R(1996), *Psychology: The Science of Mind and Behaviour*, 3rd edition, London, Hodder and Stoughton.

Grunfeld A F, Ritmillar S, Mackay K, Cowan L and Hotch D (1994), 'Detecting Domestic Violence in the Emergency Department: A Nursing Triage Model', *Journal of Emergency Nursing*, 20 (4), 271–274.

Hagemann White E (1981), in J Pahl, (ed) (1985), *Private Violence and Public Policy: The Needs of Battered Women and the Responses of the Public Services*, London, Routledge and Kegan Paul.

Hague G and Malos E (1996), *Multi-agency Responses to Domestic Violence*, Bristol, Policy Press.

Hanmer J and Maynard M (eds) (1985), *Women Violence and Social Control*, London, Macmillan.

Hart B (1986), 'Lesbian Battering, An Examination' in Kerry Lobel (ed), *Naming the Violence, Speaking Out About Lesbian Battering*, Washington, Seal Press.

Hehir B (1998), 'The Pregnancy Police', *LM*, April 1998, pp 8-9.

Heise L *et al.* (1994), 'Violence Against Women: A Neglected Public Health Issue in Less Developed Countries', *Social Science and Medicine*, 39, pp 1165-1177.

Helton A S, Anderson E and McFarlane J (1987), 'Battered and Pregnant: A Prevalence Study With Intervention Measures', *American Journal of Public Health*, 77, pp 1337-1339.

Helton A, Snodgrass F (1987), 'Batterings During Pregnancy: Intervention Strategies', *Birth*, 14, (3), pp 142-147.

Hester M, Kelly L and Radford J (eds) (1996), *Women, Violence and Male Power*, Buckingham, The Open University Press.

Hilberman E and Munson K (1978), 'Sixty Battered Women', *Victimology*, 2, pp 460-470.

Hill Collins P (1986), 'Learning from the Outsider Within: The Sociological Significance of Black Feminist Thought', *Social Problems*, 33, pp 14-32.

Hillard P A (1985), 'Physical Abuse in Pregnancy', *Obstetrics and Gynaecology*, 66, pp 185-190.

Hinde R and Stevenson-Hinde J (eds) (1973), *Constraints On Learning Limitations and Predisposition*, London, Academic Press.

Holmes T H, Rae R H (1967), 'Social readjustment rating scale', *Journal of Psychosomatic Research*, 11, pp 219–20.

Horley S (1988), *Love and Pain*, London, NCVO Publications.

Horsfall J (1991), *The Presence of the Past: Male Violence in the Family*, London, Allen and Unwin.

Hunt S C and Symonds A (1995), *The Social Meaning of Midwifery*, Basingstoke, Macmillan.

Hunt S C (2000), 'Listening to Women', Unpublished PhD Thesis, University of Warwick.

Jones L (1994), *The Social Context of Health and Health Work,* Basingstoke, Macmillan.

Joseph G (1981), 'Black Mothers and Daughters: Their Roles and Functions in American Society', in G Joseph and J Lewis (eds), *Common Differences*, Garden City, New York, Anchor.

Jukes A (1993), *Why Men Hate Women*, London, Free Association Books.

Kelly E (1986), 'Women's Experience of Sexual Violence', PhD thesis, University of Essex.

Kelly L (1988), *Surviving Sexual Violence,* London, Polity Press.

Kelly L, Regan L and Burton S (1991), 'An Exploratory Study of the Prevalence of Sexual Abuse in a Sample 1200 16-21 Year Olds', Final Report submitted to ESRC, University of North London, London.

Kelly L and Scott S (1989), 'With Our Own Hands', *Trouble and Strife*, Vol 16, pp 28-29.

Kennedy H (1992), *Eve Was Framed. Women and British Justice.* London, Chatto and Windus.

Kent A (1987), 'Home Is Where the Fear Is', *Nursing Times,* No. 85, pp 16-17.

Kingston P and Penhale B (1995) (eds), *Family Violence and the Caring Professions,* London, Macmillan.

Kohlberg L (1966), 'A Cognitive Developmental Analysis of Children's Sex Role Concepts and Attitudes', in E Maccoby (ed), *The Development of Sex Differences,* Stanford, California, Stanford University Press.

Kroll D (ed) (1996), *Midwifery Care for the Future,* London, Balliere Tindall.

Lees S (1986), *Losing Out: Sexuality and Adolescent Girls,* London, Hutchinson.

Lobel K (1986), *Naming the Violence: Speaking Out About Lesbian Battering,* Boston, MA, Seal Press.

Loizos P (1978) in Pahl J (ed) (1985), 'Private Violence and Public Policy: The Needs of Battered Women and the Responses of the Public Services', London, Routledge and Kegan Paul.

Lovenduski J and Randall V (1993), *Contemporary Feminist Politics: Women and Power,* Oxford, Oxford University Press.

Lukes S (1974), *Power: A Radical View,* Basingstoke, Macmillan.

Maccoby E E and Jacklin C N (1974), *The Psychology of Sex Differences,* California, Stanford University Press.

Mama A (1989), *The Hidden Struggle. Statutory and Voluntary Sector Responses to Violence and the Caring Professions,* London, Runnymeade Trust.

Marshall G, Newby H, Rose D and Vogler C (1988), *Social Class in Modern Britain,* London, Hutchinson.

Martin J and Roberts C (1984), *Women and Employment: A Lifetime Perspective,* London, HMSO.

Mazur A and Lamb T A (1980), 'Testosterone, Status, and Mood in Human Males', *Hormones and Behaviour,* Vol 14.

McFarlane J, Parker B, Soeken K, Bullock M (1992), 'Assessing for Abuse During Pregnancy', *Journal of the American Medical Association,* 267, pp 3176-3178.

McFarlane J, Parker B, Soeken K (1996), 'Abuse During Pregnancy: Associations With Maternal Health and Infant Birth Weight', *Nurse Research,* Jan/Feb, 45, No. 1, pp 27-41.

McGibbon A, Cooper L, Kelly L (1988), *What support?,* Child Abuse Study Unit, University of North London, London.

McRobbie A and Garber J (1977), 'Girls and Subcultures', in S Hall and T Jefferson (eds), *Resistance Through Rituals,* London, Hutchinson.

McWilliams M, McKiernan J (1993), *Bringing It Out In the Open: Women and Domestic Violence in Northern Ireland,* Belfast, HMSO.

Mead M (1935), *Sex and Temperament in Three Primitive Societies,* London, Routledge and Kegan Paul.

Mezey G C (1997), 'Domestic Violence in Pregnancy', in S Bewley, J Friend and G Mezey (eds), *Violence Against Women,* London, RCOG Press.

Mezey G C and Bewley S (1997), 'Domestic Violence and Pregnancy', *British Journal of Obstetrics and Gynaecology,* 104, pp 528-531.

Mezey G C and Bewley S (1997), 'Domestic Violence in Pregnancy', Editorial, *British Medical Journal,* Vol. 314, May.

Millett K (1970), *Sexual Politics,* London, Sphere Books.

Mooney J (1993), *The Hidden Figure: The North London Domestic Violence Survey,* Middlesex, Middlesex University Centre for Criminology.

Mullender A and Morley R (1994), *Children Living With Domestic Violence: Putting Men's Abuse of Children On the Childcare Agenda*, London, Whiting and Birch.

O'Donnell M (1988), *New Introductory Reader in Sociology*, Surrey, Thomas Nelson and Sons Ltd.

O'Hagan K and Dillenburger K (1995), *The Abuse of Women Within Child Care Work*, Buckingham, Open University Press.

Oakley A (1985), *Sex, Gender and Society*, Aldershot, Gower.

Office for National Statistics (1996), *Social Trends 26*, London, The Stationery Office.

Ogg J and Bennett G (1992), 'Screening for Elder Abuse in the Community', *Geriatric Medicine*, February, pp 63-67.

Okely J (1983), *The Traveller-Gypsies*, Cambridge, Cambridge University Press.

Olweus D, Mattsson A, Schallin D and Low H (1980), 'Testosterone, Aggression, Physical and Personality Dimensions', in 'Normal Adolescent Males', *Psychosomatic Medicine*, vol 42.

Pahl J (ed) (1985), *Private Violence and Public Policy: The Needs of Battered Women and the Responses of the Public Services*, London, Routledge and Kegan Paul.

Painter K (1991), *Wife Rape and the Law Survey Report: Key Findings and Recommendations*, Department of Social Policy and Social Work, University of Manchester, Manchester, England.

Paluzzi P A and Slattery L (1996), *No Woman Deserves to Hurt. Domestic Violence Education for Women's Health Care Providers*, USA, American College of Nurse-Midwives.

Parker B, McFarlane J and Soeken K (1994), 'Abuse During Pregnancy: Effects On Maternal Complications and Birth Weights in Adult and Teenage Women', *Obstetrics and Gynaecology*, No. 84, pp 323-328.

Parkes C M (1975), *Bereavement: Studies of Grief in Adult Life*, Harmondsworth, Penguin.

Pearson R (1992), 'Looking Both Ways: Extending the Debate On Women and Citizenship in Europe' in A Ward, J Gregory and N Yuval Davis (eds), *Women and Citizenship in Europe*, Stoke on Trent, Trentham Books.

Persky H, Smith K D and Basu G K (1971), 'Relation of Psychologic Measures of Aggression and Hostility to Testosterone Production in Man', *Psychosomatic Medicine*, vol 33.

Plichta S (1992), 'The Effects of Woman Abuse on Health Care Utilization and Health Status: A Review of the Literature', *Women's Health Institute*, 2, No. 3, Fall 1992, pp 154–163.

Prochaska J O, DiClemente C C, Velicer W F, Rosser J S (1993), 'Standardized, Individualized, Interactive and Personalized Self Help Programs for Smoking Cessation', *Health Psychology*, 12, pp 399-405.

Radford J (1987), 'Policing Male Violence, Policing Women', in J Hanmer and M Maynard (eds), *Women, Violence and Social Control*, Basingstoke, Macmillan.

Radford L, Hester M and Pearson C (1998), *Domestic Violence Fact Sheet*, Women's Aid Federation, Bristol.

Rheingold H and Cook K (1975), 'The Contents of Boys' and Girls' Rooms as an Index of Parents' Behaviour', *Child Development*, part 46, pp 459–463.

Robinson J (1996), 'The Battered Fetus', *British Journal of Midwifery*, September, 4, No. 9, pp 496-498.

Roldan M (1982) in J Pahl (ed) (1985), *Private Violence and Public Policy: The Needs of Battered Women and the Responses of the Public Services*, London, Routledge and Kegan Paul.

Rose D and O'Reilly K (1997), *Constructing Classes Towards a New Social Classification for the UK*, Swindon, ESRC Office of National Statistics.

Royal College of Midwives (1997), 'Domestic Abuse in Pregnancy', Position Paper Number 19, November, Cardiff, Royal College of Midwives.

Rubin J Z, Provenzano F J and Luria Z (1974), 'The Eye of the Beholder: Parents' Views on the Sex of New Borns', *American Journal of Orthopsychiatry*.

Russell D (1982), *Rape in Marriage*, New York, Macmillan.

Russell D (1984), *Sexual Exploitation*, Beverly Hills, CA, Sage.

Russell D (1985), *Incest. The Secret Trauma*, New York, Basic Books.

Russell D (1993), *Making Violence Sexy. Feminist Views on Pornography*, Buckingham, Open University Press.

Salzman L E (1990), 'Battering During Pregnancy: A Role for Physicians', *Atlanta Medicine*, 65, pp 45-48.

Saradjian J (1999), *The Yorkshire Post*, 9 June 1999.

Sassetti M R (1993), 'Domestic Violence' in B A Elliott, M D Halverson and M Hendricks-Mathews (Guest eds), *Primary Care*, 20, No. 2, pp 289-306.

Satin A J, Ramin S M, Paicurich J (1992), 'The Prevalence of Sexual Assault: A Survey of 2404 Puerperal Women', *American Journal of Obstetrics and Gynecology*, 167, No. 4, Part 1, pp 973-975.

Saunders C (1982), in J Pahl (ed) (1985), *Private Violence and Public Policy: The Needs of Battered Women and the Responses of the Public Services*, London, Routledge and Kegan Paul.

Schei B and Bakketeig (1989), 'Gynaecological Impact of Sexual and Physical Abuse by Spouse. A Study of a Random Sample of Norweigian Women', *British Journal of Obstetrics and Gynaecology*, 6, pp 1379–1383

Schlegel von F (1972) in J Pahl (ed) (1985), *Private Violence and Public Policy: The Needs of Battered Women and the Responses of the Public Services*, London, Routledge and Kegan Paul.

Schornstein S (1997), *Domestic Violence and Healthcare: What Every Professional Needs To Know*, New York, Sage Publications.

Scott S (1994), 'Lies, Lesbians and Statistics', *Trouble and Strife*, 28, pp 36-40.

Sears J (1992), 'Uptake of Science 'A' Levels: an ICI and BP sponsored project for ASE Education in Science', 149:30.

Skelton C (1993), 'Women and Education', in D Richardson and V Robinson (eds), *Introducing Women's Studies: Feminising Theory and Practice*, London, Macmillan.

Smith L J F (1989), *Domestic Violence: An Overview of the Literature*, Home Office Research Study No. 107, London, HMSO.

Spender D (1982), *Women Of Ideas - And What Men Have Done To Them*, London, Unwin Hyman.

Stainton Rogers W (1991), *Explaining Health and Illness: On Exploring Adversity*, London, Harvester Wheatsheaf.

Stanko E (1985), *Intimate Intrusions*, London, Unwin Hyman.

Stanko E (1990), *Everyday Violence*, London, Pandora.

Stanko E (1992), 'Wife Battering: All in the Family' in A Giddens (ed), *Human Societies*, Cambridge, Polity.

Stanko E, Crisp D, Hale C and Lucraft H (1997), *Counting the Costs: Estimating the Impact of Domestic Violence in the London Borough of Hackney*, Swindon, Crime Concern.

Stark E, Flitcraft A, Frazier W (1979), 'Medicine and Patriarchal Violence: The Social Construction of a 'Private' Event', *International Journal of Health Service*, 9, pp 461-93.

Stark E, Flitcraft A (1996), *Women At Risk*, London, Sage.

Statistics Canada (1996), *Survey On Violence Against Women in Canada*, Canada, Statistics Canada.

Stewart D and Cecutti A (1993), 'Physical Abuse in Pregnancy', *Journal of the Canadian Medical Association*, 149, No. 9, pp 1257-1263.

Stewart D E (1994), 'Incidence of Postpartum Abuse in Women With a History of Abuse During Pregnancy', *Journal of the Canadian Medical Association*, 151, No. 11, pp 1601-1604.

Strauss A, Gelles R J and Steinmetz S K (1980), *Violence Behind Closed Doors: Violence in the American Family*, New York, Anchor Books.

Sutherland C, Bybee D, Sullivan C (1998), 'The Long Term Effects of Battering on Women's Health', *Women's Health: Research on Gender, Behaviour and Policy*, No. 4, pp 41-70, Lawrence Erlbaum Associates.

Taylor J and Chandler T (1995), *Lesbians Talk: Violent Relationships*, London, Scarlet Press.

Townsend P and Davidson N (1986), *The Black Report. Inequalities in Health*, Harmondsworth, Penguin.

Townsend P, Whitehead M and Davidson N (eds) (1992), *Inequalities in Health: The Black Report and the Health Divide* (New Edition), Harmondsworth, Penguin.

UKCC (United Kingdom Central Council for Nursing, Midwifery and Health Visiting), *1998 Guidelines for Records and Record Keeping*.

UKCC (United Kingdom Central Council for Nursing, Midwifery and Health Visiting), *1998 Midwives Rules and Code of Practice*.

Victim Support (1996), *Women, Rape, and the Criminal Justice System*, London, Victim Support.

Walby S (1990), *Theorising Patriarchy*, London, Blackwell.

Walker I. (1984), *The Battered Women's Syndrome*, New York, Springer.

Watson L (1996), *Victims of Violent Crime*

Recorded by the Police 1990-1994, Home Office Statistical Findings, http://www.homeoffice.gov.uk/cpd/cpsu/domviol98.htm

Webster J, Chandler J and Battisutta D (1996), 'Pregnancy Outcomes and Health Care Use – The Effects of Abuse', *American Journal of Obstetrics and Gynecology*, 174, pp 760-767.

Webster J, Sweett S, Stolz T A (1994), 'Domestic Violence in Pregnancy: A Prevalence Study', *Medical Journal of Australia*, 161, pp 466-471.

Whitehead M (1988), *The Health Divide*, London, Penguin.

Whittaker T (1996), 'Violence, Gender and Elder Abuse' in B Fawcett *et al.*, *Violence and Gender Relations*, London, Sage Publications.

Wilkinson G, Miers M (eds) (1999), *Power and Nursing Practice*, Macmillan Press, London.

Wilson E (1983), *What Is To Be Done About Violence Towards Women?* Harmondsworth, Penguin.

Wollstonecraft M (1982/1792), *Vindication of the Rights of Woman*, Harmondsworth, Penguin.

Yeandle S (1984), *Women's Working Lives: Patterns and Strategies*, London, Tavistock.

Young A and McFarlane J (1991), 'Preventing Abuse During Pregnancy: A National Educational Model for Health Providers', *Journal of Nurse Education*, 30, pp 202-6.

Index